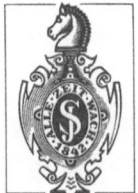

Progress in Pediatric Surgery

Volume 25

Co-founding Editor
P. P. Rickham

Editors
T. A. Angerpointner
M. W. L. Gauderer · W. Ch. Hecker
J. Prévot · L. Spitz
U. G. Stauffer · P. Wurnig

Operative Technique in Neonates and Infants

Volume Editor

T. A. Angerpointner, Munich

With 77 Figures, some in color
and 34 Tables

Springer-Verlag Berlin Heidelberg GmbH

Priv.-Doz. Dr. THOMAS A. ANGERPOINTNER
Zenettistraße 48/III, D-8000 Munich 2
Federal Republic of Germany

Volumes 1–17 of this series were published
by Urban & Schwarzenberg, Baltimore–Munich

ISBN 978-3-642-87709-4   ISBN 978-3-642-87707-0 (eBook)
DOI 10.1007/978-3-642-87707-0

Library of Congress Cataloging-in-Publication Data
Operative technique in neonates and infants /
volume editor, Th. A. Angerpointner.   p.   cm. – (Progress in pediatric surgery; v. 25)
Includes bibliographical references.

1. Infants (Newborn) – Surgery. 2. Infants – Surgery. 3. Surgery, Operative.
[1. Surgery, Operative – in infancy & childhood.]
I. Angerpointner, Thomas. II. Series.
[DNLM: W1 PR677KA v. 25 / WO 925 O61]   RD137.A1P7   vol. 25   [RD137.5]
617.9′8 s – dc20   [617.9′8]   DNLM/DLC   89-21793

Typesetting and printing: Petersche Druckerei, Rothenburg ob der Tauber

2123/3145-543210   Printed on acid-free paper

Contents

Editors

Angerpointner, T. A., Priv.-Doz. Dr.
Zenettistraße 48/III, D-8000 München 2

Gauderer, Michael, W. L., MD
University Pediatric Surgical Associates, 2101 Adelbert Road
Cleveland, OH 44106, USA

Hecker, W. Ch., Prof. Dr.
Kinderchirurgische Klinik im Dr. von Haunerschen Kinderspital
der Universität München, Lindwurmstraße 4
D-8000 München 2

Prévot, J., Prof.
Clinique Chirurgical Pédiatrique, Hôpital d'Enfants de Nancy
F-54511 Vandœvre Cedex

Rickham, P. P., Prof. Dr.
MD, MS, FRCS, FRCSI, FRACS, DCH, FAAP
Universitätskinderklinik, Chirurgische Abteilung
Steinwiesstraße 75, CH-8032 Zürich

Spitz, L., Prof., PhD, FRCS, Nuffield Professor of Pediatric Surgery
Institute of Child Health, University of London
Hospital for Sick Children, Great Ormond Street, 30 Guilford Street
GB-London WC1N 1EH

Stauffer, U. G., Prof. Dr.
Universitätskinderklinik, Kinderchirurgische Abteilung
Steinwiesstraße 75, CH-8032 Zürich

Wurnig, P., Prof. Dr.
Kinderchirurgische Abteilung des
Mautner Markhof'schen Kinderspitals
Baumgasse 75, A-1030 Wien

Contributors

You will find the addresses at the beginning of the respective contribution

Angerpointner, T. A.   1, 32
Berlien, H. P.   5
Deltz, E.   90
Dohrmann, P.   97, 132
Gdanietz, K.   68
Geissler, W.   58
Gerhard, A.   71
Hamelmann, H.   90
Hedenborg, L.   48
Heller, K.   81
Hoffecker, A.   32
Holschneider, A. M.   103
Kellenberger, R.   123
Körner, K.   58
Koltai, J. L.   71
Lauterjung, K. L.   32

Mengel, W.   90, 97, 132
Müller, G.   5
Noack, L.   68
Schaube, H.   97
Schmittenbecher, P. P.   23
Stauffer, U. G.   39
Thomasson, B.   48
Urban, A. E.   118
von Laer, L.   123
Vorpahl, K.   68
Waag, K. L.   81
Waldschmidt, J.   5
Wiksell, H.   48
Wit, J.   68
Wurnig, P.   58

Dedication

In Honor of Professor Waldemar Christian Hecker

Professor Waldemar Christian Hecker celebrated his 65th birthday on 15 February 1987. He received cordial congratulations from friends and colleagues from all over the world. On this occasion, a symposium on "Operative Technique in Neonates and Infants" was organized by his students and associates.

Together with P. P. Rickham of Zurich and J. Prevot of Nancy, W. C. Hecker initiated the series *Progress in Pediatric Surgery* in 1970, which was published first by Urban and Schwarzenberg and, since 1985, by Springer. So far, 25 volumes on different aspects and problems in paediatric surgery have been published under a distinguished editorial board. Volume 25 of *Progress in Pediatric Surgery* is in honor of Professor Hecker on his 65th birthday. Some excellent papers presented at the birthday symposium were chosen for publication in this volume; which also contains other, invited contributions.

Some landmarks in Professor Hecker's life may be briefly mentioned. Waldemar Christian Hecker was born on 15 February 1922 in Potsdam near Berlin. Early in his life he was introduced to surgery by his father, himself a surgeon-in-chief. Following World War II he studied medicine in Hamburg and passed his medical exams in 1950. He obtained his doctor's degree by studies on treatment of skull base fractures in 1951. Konjetzny and Linder were his main surgical teachers, leading him to paediatric surgery, in Germany then still a very young subspeciality of general surgery. In 1962 he wrote his PhD thesis on *Problems and Clinical Aspects of Congenital Atresias of the Digestive Tract.* Under the guidance of Linder, who took him from Berlin to Heidelberg, Hecker established a paediatric surgical division at the University Surgical Hospital of Heidelberg in 1963. He became Professor of Paediatric Surgery in 1967 and succeeded Professor Anton Oberniedermayr as Ordinarius of Paediatric Surgery at the University of Munich in 1969, the first regular chair of paediatric surgery in Germany.

Owing to his scientific activities and his medical practice, Professor Hecker soon acquired an international reputation. He played a major role in establishing paediatric surgery as an independent discipline in Germany. He was and is a member of many committees of the General Medical Council, has been President of the German Society of Paediatric Surgery, President of the Bavarian Association of General Surgeons, and was honoured with the Cross of Merit of the Federal Republic of Germany. More than 300 publications, many contributions to paediatric surgical and paediatric handbooks, and two books *(Elementary Pediatric Surgery* and *Surgical Correction of the Intersexual and the Malformed External Female Genitalia)* document Professor Hecker's active interests in numerous topics of paediatric surgery.

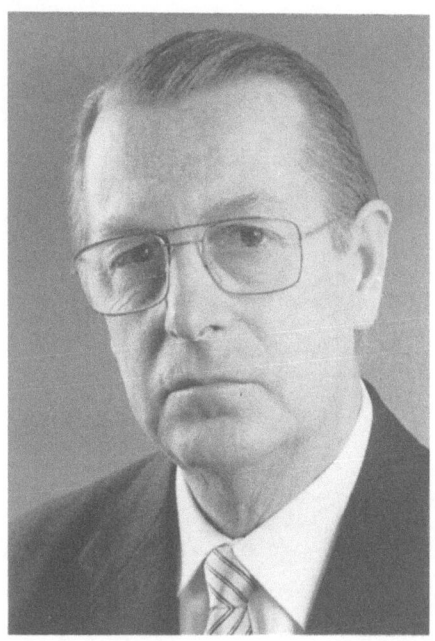

The Editorial Board of *Progress in Pediatric Surgery* expresses its thanks to Professor Hecker by dedicating this volume to him on his 65th birthday, wishing him many happy and active years crowned with the success we have come to associate with his name.

THOMAS A. ANGERPOINTNER

Portrait-photograph: Doris Feder, Dr. von Haunersches Kinderspital of the University of Munich

Lasers in Pediatric Surgery

H. P. Berlien[1,2], G. Müller[2], and J. Waldschmidt[3]

Summary

During the last few years the laser has become a very interesting instrument in pediatric surgery. This is the result of the wide variation in tissue interactions and the possibility of specific applications. The CO_2 laser is a highly precise cutting instrument whereas the argon laser has its great advantage in the treatment of superficial vascular anomalies. The most important laser in pediatric surgery is the Nd:YAG laser, on the one hand because its radiation can be transmitted by fibres, on the other because with the relationship between interaction time and power density, and the choice of application, it is possible to change the tissue interaction from precise cutting to specific coagulation and homogeneous coagulation. As a result, indications for lasers in pediatric surgery range from the treatment of superficial haemangiomas to typical endoscopic procedures and the resection of parenchymatous organs and tumours.

Zusammenfassung

Der Laser ist in den letzten Jahren zu einem interessanten Instrument in der Kinderchirurgie geworden, und zwar aufgrund der großen Variationsbreite der Wechselwirkungen mit einzelnen Gewebearten und der Möglichkeit spezifischer Anwendungen. Der CO_2-Laser ist ein Präzisionsschneideinstrument, während der Argon-Laser besonders bei der Behandlung oberflächlicher vaskulärer Anomalien Vorteile bietet. Der wichtigste Laser in der Kinderchirurgie ist der Neodym-Yag-Laser, da einerseits die Lichtstrahlung durch Glasfasern übertragbar ist und da andererseits aufgrund variabler Einwirkzeit, Leistungsdichte und Applikationsart verschiedene Anwendungsmöglichkeiten bestehen: vom präzisen Schneiden bis zur Punkt- und Flächenkoagulation. Daraus läßt sich für den Laser in der Kinderchirurgie eine Indikationsliste erstellen, die von der Behandlung oberflächlicher und tiefer kavernöser Hämangiome über alle gängigen endoskopischen Verfahren bis zur Resektion parenchymatöser Organe und Tumoren reicht.

Résumé

Le laser est devenu, au cours de ces dernières années, un instrument de choix en chirurgie infantile. Cela est dû à la gamme très étendue des interactions obtenues avec certains tissus et au fait que l'application peut être parfaitement spécifique. Le laser au CO_2 est un instrument tranchant d'une extrême précision alors que le laser Argon est plus efficace pour le traitement des anomalies vasculaires superficielles. Le laser le plus important en chirurgie infantile est le laser Neodym-Yag car, d'une part le faisceau émis peut être transmis par des fibres de verre et d'autre part, vu que l'on peut varier à volonté le temps d'action, la puissance volumique et le mode d'applica-

[1]Department of Laser Medicine, [2]Laser-Medizin-Zentrum GmbH, Berlin and [3]Pediatric Surgical Department, Klinikum Steglitz, Freie Universität Berlin, Hindenburgdamm 30, D-1000 Berlin 45, Federal Republic of Germany

Progress in Pediatric Surgery, Vol. 25
Angerpointner (Ed.)
© Springer-Verlag Berlin Heidelberg 1990

tion, il peut être utilisé pour obtenir des incisions nettes ou encore des coagulations ponctuelles ou en surface. Le laser est donc la technique de choix dans un grand nombre de cas, qu'il s'agisse du traitement d'hémangiomes superficiels du caverneux ou de toutes les techniques d'endoscopies courantes ou encore de résection d'organes parenchymateux ou de tumeurs.

Physical Basis of Laser Medicine

Laser is an acronym for light amplification by stimulated emission of radiation. This phenomenon was first postulated by Einstein in 1917 [9], whereby the atoms or molecules of a suitable material are excited to a higher energy level by energy pumping (Fig. 1). The most important active media are:

Gases (e.g. noble gases or their ions, molecular gases or vapours)
Fluids (e.g. organic dyes in solution)
Solids (e.g. crystals and glasses doped with metal atoms and/or rare earths)
Semiconductor elements (laser diodes)

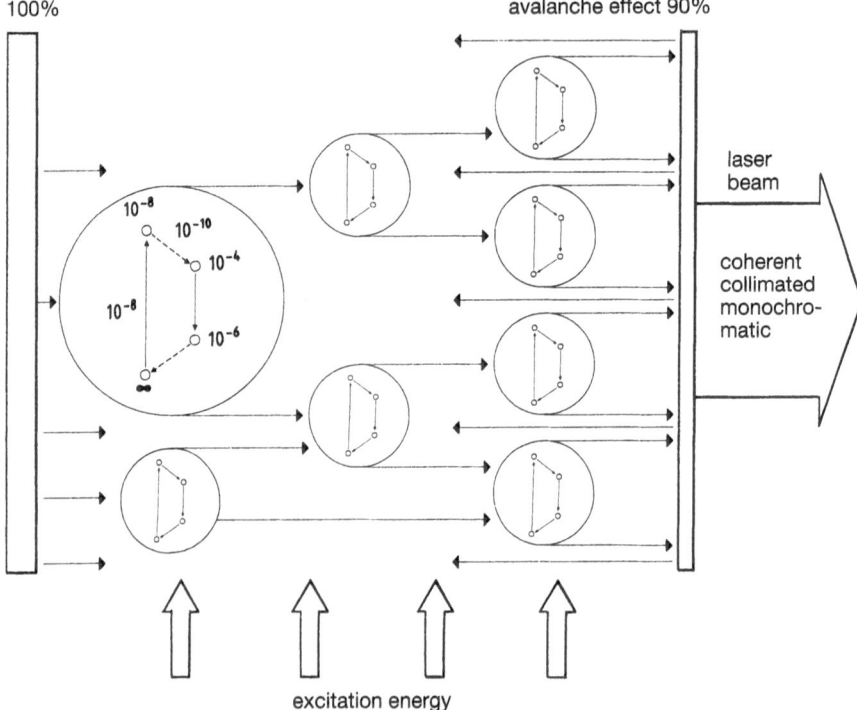

Fig. 1. Energy pumping. If an atom or molecule is excited (*left-hand side* of the diagram) and an additional photon with appropriate frequency impinges on an excited system, this is forced into resonance and a second, identical photon is released when the system reverts to the lower energy state (*central part* of the diagram). Between a highly reflecting and semitransparent mirror the photons are reflected back and forth and stimulate other excited systems to release resonance photos, thus generating an avalanche effect (*right-hand side* of the diagram)

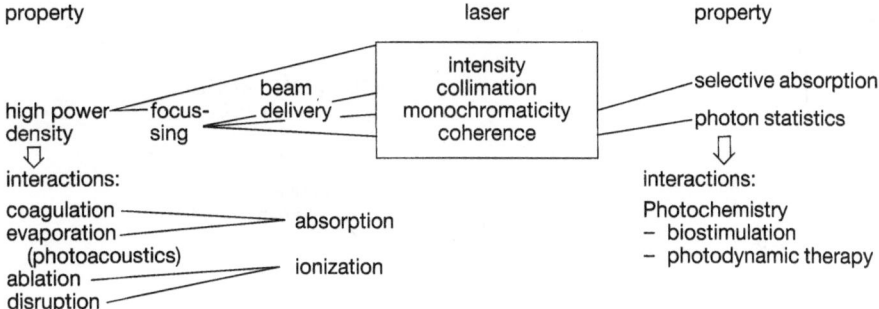

Fig. 2. Interdependence of the physical properties of the laser and the tissue interactions used in medicine

The energy supply, the so-called pumping, results from:

Electrical gas discharge
Chemical reaction
Electromagnetic radiation within the radio frequency and optical range
Electric current

The laser differs from the thermal light sources, as represented by an incandescent lamp, in three characteristic properties which are important for medical treatment:

1. Coherence. Individual rays within a light beam have a certain spatial and temporal relationship (constant phase).
2. Collimation. Laser radiation forms a beam with almost no divergence, i.e. the rays are parallel to one another.
3. Monochromaticity. Only a narrow spectral band of high intensity is emitted, i.e. it is extremely monochromatic.

These three characteristics make it possible to focus a laser beam into a very small cross-sectional area and thereby to reach very high energy densities (Fig. 2), thus offering treatment with high precision and without mechanical force.

Just a few months after the discovery of the first laser by Maiman, physicians in the United States began to get interested in using this new source of light. This is not surprising as therapy with light was already well established. Today we differentiate between three principal classes of interaction.

Laser-Tissue Interaction

The effectiveness of radiation with different kinds of tissue is mainly determined by two parameters [7]. These are, first, the interaction time of the radiation with the tissue, and, second, the effective energy density, whereby the specific absorption of the tissue must be taken into consideration (Fig. 3). At lower energy densi-

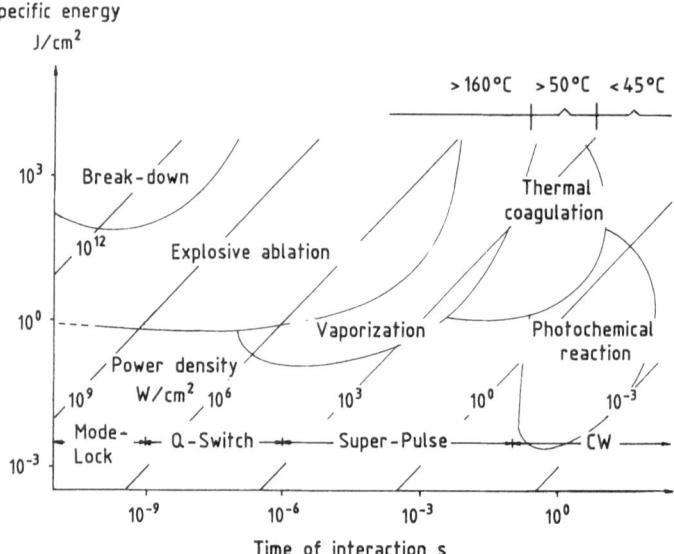

Fig. 3. Photochemical reactions occur with a long exposure time and low energy and nonlinear interactions with short pulses and a high specific energy. Between them is the large area of thermal interactions

ties, with a long reaction time, photochemical processes occur by absorption of light, which does not primarily lead to heating of the tissue. An example is the light-induced photochemical reaction of artificial chromophores. According to our present knowledge, biostimulation should also be considered a photochemical effect.

With decreasing interaction time and higher energy densities in the transition region to photocoagulation, we enter the domain of photothermally induced effects. At temperatures between 40° and 50°C cell membranes are relaxed, the cells swell, and protein fibrils migrate out of the cells. When the tissues cool down, they adhere to each other, thus fusing neighbouring cells. This effect can be utilized for tissue welding.

Thermic dynamic reactions also belong to this transition area. In this case the thermal events described lead to an inflammatory reaction which is followed by a reorganization of the irradiated tissue. The resulting repair leads to the desired effect within a few weeks. This effect is currently used in the therapy of port-wine stains, spider naevi, superficial angiomatoses and also for keloid treatment. Even the "photocoagulation" used in ophthalmology belongs to this type of interaction. In the case of a retina detachment, the retina should be fixed to the base, leaving the nutritive vessels unaffected.

At temperatures between 60° and 100°C denaturation and coagulation occur. Although the near-infrared radiation of the Nd:YAG laser is relatively strongly absorbed by haemoglobin and melanin, it penetrates rather homogeneously into the tissue. As a result the depth of penetration is approximately 5 mm. This leads to a homogeneous volume coagulation, which is used for haemostasis and tumour denaturation. The Nd:YAG laser also achieves higher energy densities, so that tissues heat to over 100°C with vaporization of water and resulting dessication. When this point is reached, the tissue itself is vaporized very quickly. This allows larger areas of tumour tissue to be removed and tissue to be cut (Table 1).

For lasers with less penetration depth, for example the CO_2 laser, all the irradiation is absorbed on the surface so we very soon reach a temperature of more than 200°C. This immediately produces vaporization of the tissue, with a cutting effect. Owing to the minimal penetration depth and short exposure times, thermal conductivity is not very important and the coagulation border is small. Thus precise cuts for microsurgical procedures can be made (Fig. 4).

Table 1. Damage caused by thermal laser irradiation

Temperature (C)	Tissue interaction
≤ 40°	No irreversible tissue damage
40°–45°	Enzyme induction, oedema, membrane swelling and, depending on time, cell death
60°	Protein denaturation, coagulation and necrosis
80°	Collagen denaturation, membrane defect
100°	Drying
> 150°	Carbonization
> 300°	Vaporization

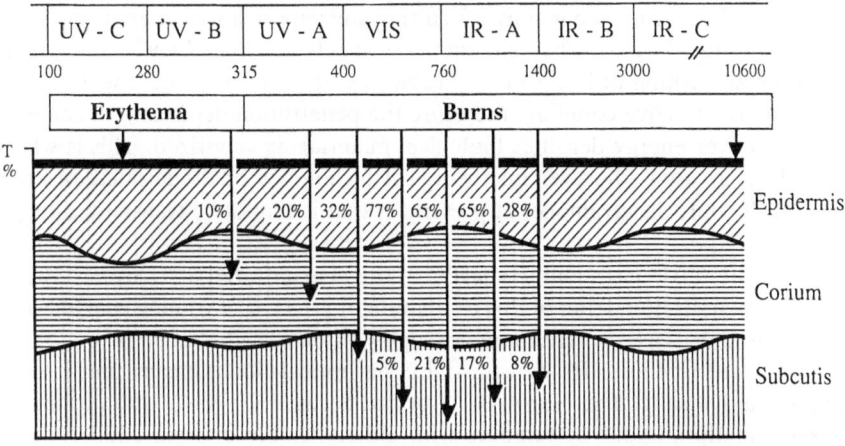

Fig. 4. Light intensity as a function of depth and wavelength in human skin (the intensity at the surface is assumed to be 100%)

As the light intensity increases, the electromagnetic nature of light, with its coupled oscillating electrical and magnetical fields, becomes more important. At very high light intensities the electrical fields that are produced can be large enough to ionize the atoms and molecules of the air, i.e. to remove the electrons from the positive core [8]. In physics one speaks of the formation of plasma, as occurs within sparks. This is called optical breakdown, but before optical breakdown occurs, the field strength passes through a domain which does not involve complete ionization, but where the photon density and the associated field strength are already very high. Here the structures of molecules or crystal lattices are disrupted. This is called photoablation or photodesorption, as it is possible in this intensity region to etch surfaces by light without thermal side effects.

In the transition area between the thermal effects of absorption and the effects of ionization, we have the so-called photoacoustic interaction. The absorption of short light pulses leads to a heating of the target tissue, which results in thermal expansion. In the case of repetitive pulses an oscillating density change is induced and, depending on the pulse frequency, an acoustic thermal wave is generated which applies mechanical stress and strain to the target tissue and may lead to rupture as the desired effect.

Laser Systems in Medicine

The most important medical lasers with their fields of application are shown in Table 2. Besides the argon laser, which is used because of its high selectivity for natural chromophores (e.g. haemoglobin), the argon ion pumped dye laser is also gaining in importance [5]. It enables one to cover a larger spectral range, from blue-green to the red end of the spectrum. This is not only interesting for a whole range of natural chromophores (with improved selectivity), but also for synthetic chromophores which may be coupled to other substances, if necessary.

The CO_2 laser is used mainly for cutting and vaporization. It emits in the mid-infrared ($9.6-10.6\,\mu m$). The light energy is mainly absorbed by water. Compared with the absorption of lasers in the visible, we are concerned here with a $10-100$ times more effective coupling; therefore the penetration depth is very small, and even at lower energy densities biological materials is vaporized. This is why the CO_2 laser is used wherever microsurgical techniques or tissue ablation are required. Its only disadvantage, at present, is that it cannot be transmitted by optical fibres [6].

The Nd:YAG laser emits typically in the near-infrared at $1.06\,\mu m$. Owing to the high penetration depth of this irradiation, it is a typical volume coagulator and is used in those cases where there are highly vascularized structures, e.g. malformations and tumours. Its transmissivity via optical fibres means that it can be applied universally. The Nd:YAG laser can be used for coagulation of haemorrhages, malformations or tumours with either flexible or rigid endoscopes. At higher energy it may also be used for recanalization of tumour stenoses or even vascular obstructions. With a handpiece and corresponding high energy density,

Table 2. Laser in medicine

Type	Mode	Wavelength (μm)	Power (W)	Characteristics	Effect	Use		Medical fields
						Coagulation	Cutting	
Ar^+	cw	0.488, 0.514	2–10	Specific absorption by haemoglobin and melanin	Coagulation	+		Surgery, urology, dermatology, ENT, ophthalmology
Argon dye	cw	0.488–0.788	0.5–3	Specific absorption by natural and synthetic chromophores	Coagulation	(+)		Plastic surgery, dermatology, oncology, ophthalmology
Nd:YAG	cw	1.06	10–120	Volume absorption	Coagulation	++	+	Surgery, urology, dermatology, neurosurgery, gastroenterology, pulmonology
Nd:YAG	pulsed	1.06	1 MW per pulse	Optomechanical effect	Photodisruption		++	Ophthalmology
CO_2	cw	10.6	20–60	High absorption by water	Cutting	(+)	++	Surgery, urology, dermatology, gynaecology, neurosurgery, ENT, maxillofacial surgery

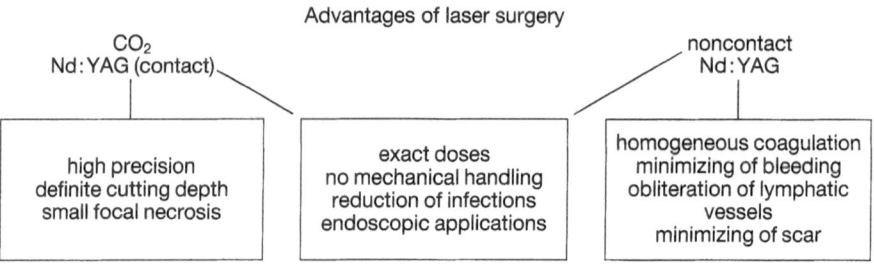

Fig. 5. Typical properties and advantages of the two most important surgical lasers

the resection of parenchymatous organs with simultaneous haemostasis is possible.

Pulsed Nd: YAG laser systems are used in ophthalmology for the treatment of the posterior capsular membrane as well as in the surgery of glaucoma.

The advantages of the laser in medicine can be summarized as follows (Fig. 5):

1. Haemostasis
2. High precision
3. Reduced instrumentation at the treatment site
4. Non-contact tissue removal: asepsis (no contamination)
5. Minimal trauma to the surrounding tissue (no mechanical forces applied)

Fields of Application

Independent of the type of laser-tissue interaction and of medical specialty, it is possible to define different fields of application of laser treatment (Table 3).

Table 3. The principal fields of application for lasers in medicine

Surface	Skin, visible mucosa, cornea
Vascular diseases	Venous arterial
Endoscopy	Natural ostia, cavities
Open surgery	Cavities and organs, soft tissue, orthopaedics

Surface

As is to be expected, most of the indications of this kind are found in the field of dermatology. However it is also used in surgery, in particular in plastic surgery, urology, gynaecology and ophthalmology (e.g. corneal surgery). The argon and the argon pumped dye lasers are suited for the treatment of pigmentation anomalies. Even the Nd: YAG laser is used here with success. For large lesions, the CO_2

laser can be used for vaporization, but it is also possible to achieve limited depth coagulation with the argon and Nd:YAG lasers [1].

Haemangiomas are the most frequent malformations in childhood, and their treatment is controversial. Most haemangiomas heal spontaneously before the age of 8, and it is advisable to wait till then. If the haemangioma is located at an exposed position, e.g. on the face or on functionally important structures, further growth can result in significant functional disorders or disfigurement. This requires early treatment in infancy and childhood (Table 4).

Until now all treatment methods have been radical and have caused further injury. One prominent example is X-ray therapy. After a period of 20–30 years

Table 4. Indications for laser therapy in angiomas[a]

Rapid growth with spread to mucous membranes and conjunctiva

Functional disorders with occlusion of lumina and destruction or organs (pharynx, larynx, trachea, and bronchi)

Exulceration, superinfection and bleeding

Gastrointestinal bleeding

Arteriovenous shunts with cardiac disease or steal phenomenon

Preoperative volume reduction

Angiomas of parenchymatous organs

Cosmetic correction

[a] Owing to the spontaneous healing of angiomas the indications for laser therapy are very strong. Only these indications need early laser therapy

Table 5. Types of angiomas and preferred lasers for therapy

Angiomatosis	Ar^+	Ar^+ dye	Nd:YAG non-contact	Nd:YAG contact	CO_2
Spider naevi	++		+		
Port-wine stain	++		(+)		
Cutaneous haemangioma					
Strawberry	++		++		
Cavernous			++	++	
Combined	+		++	++	
Angioma (cavernoma)					
Resection			++	++	
Volume reduction			++	++	
Vascular hamartia			++	+	
Haemangioendothelioma			++	+	
Venectasia				++	
Telangiectasia	++		+		
Varices				+	

treatment can result in the development of malignancy. The initial hopes in using lasers have not always been fulfilled, especially regarding cosmetic results in children. Treatment has been carried out almost entirely with the argon laser. This radiation is strongly absorbed by haemoglobin, permitting selective treatment of vessel anomalies (Table 5).

Since 1983 we have used the argon laser. Early instruments offered relatively low power (2–3 W output) with long pulse duration (0.1 s). Thermal skin damage was not always avoidable. Further development of instrumental technique allowed increased selectivity for haemoglobin with an output of 5–6 W, exposure times of 0.02 s and minimization of heat conduction by the short exposure time. With this technique one can successfully treat plain and strawberry haemangiomas, spider naevi and port-wine stains. Because of the good experience with high selectivity and a minimum of wound pain caused by the short exposure time, we start treatment in childhood. This is very important as children with these conditions are often treated badly by other children during play. General anaesthesia is very seldom necessary. Normally sedation and local anaesthesia are sufficient. In order to avoid scars it is important not to induce coagulation of the irradiation area during treatment, but to induce the so-called thermic dynamic reaction which occurs spontaneously within 3–4 weeks. Therefore the second session should not occur within the next 4–6 weeks. Normally we wait 8–12 weeks (Table 6).

Because of the high selectivity of absorption by haemoglobin, the argon laser is not useful for the treatment of larger vessel anomalies. For treatment of these larger and more deeply situated anomalies the Nd:YAG laser is preferred, owing to its relatively high penetration depth (Table 7). Conventional applications still caused skin burns, and these treatments have therefore been abandoned. Procedures for skin cooling with chlorethyl or saline solution did not give sufficient protection.

Table 6. Treatment of superficial lesions with the argon laser (0.48, 0.51 μm)

Power	5 W
Spot size	0.5 mm
Pulse duration	0.02 s
Repetition rate	6/s
Remarks	Prevent surface coagulation, late thermodynamic sequelae, period of treatment 8 weeks

Table 7. Treatment of intradermal parts of combined vessel anomalies with the Nd:YAG laser (10.6 μm)

Power	20 W
Spot size	1.5 mm
Pulse duration	0.05 s
Repetition rate	6/s
Remarks	Prevent visual surface coagulation, thermodynamic late sequelae, period of treatment 8 weeks

6 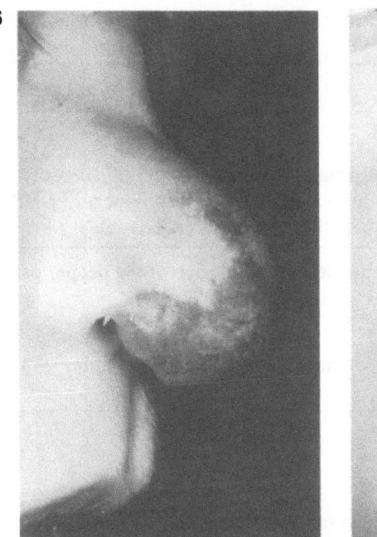 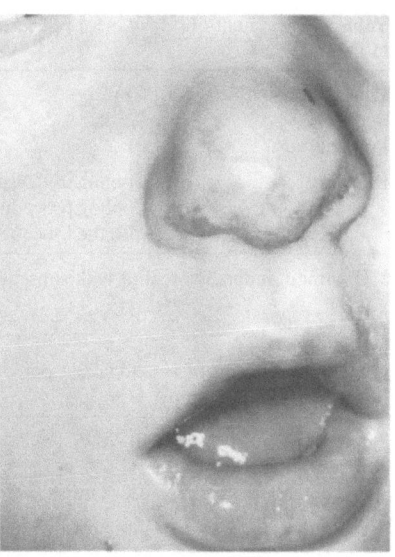 7

Fig. 6. Combined tuberous and cavernous haemangioma of the nose (preoperative)

Fig. 7. After two treatments with transcutaneous Nd:YAG laser irradiation and ice cube cooling: regression and blanching of the angioma

Because the transmission of the near-infrared radiation of the Nd:YAG laser in water is quite high, efficient surface cooling can be obtained by using ice cubes. Conventionally produced ice cubes have substantial air occlusions, which can lead to dispersion of the irradiation. These ice cubes should not be used. Ice cubes made by ice machines near 0°C and under high pressure have scarcely any air occlusions and are almost crystal clear. Because of residual absorption and dispersion, an output of about 50 W is necessary. Furthermore, the ice cube has to make good contact with the skin. Otherwise skin burns will occur. Another important effect is the compression of the haemangioma caused by the ice cube, so that the blood is partially pressed out, improving irradiation of the vessel walls, and irradiation can penetrate deeper into the tissue [4]. With this procedure large haemangiomas can be treated and made to regress (Figs. 6 and 7). For partial remissions it is possible to resect previously inoperable angiomas (Table 8).

Another application is percutaneous intraluminal irradiation of larger cavernomas by the bare fibre (Table 9). After puncture of the angioma with a special cannula the fibre is introduced into the vascular lumen [2]. With an output of 10–20 W and slow withdrawal of the fibre, the vessel is irradiated at a rate of 0.2–1 mm/s. Continuous rinsing of the fibre tip with NaCl solution prevents destruction of the fibre by adherent blood and thrombus formation, so that radiation can reach the vessel wall with subsequent vasculitis and obliteration. Even with this procedure a volume reduction can be achieved, so that previously inoperable angiomas can be resected. The Nd:YAG laser has proved effective for

Table 8. Treatment of subcutaneous parts of combined vessel anomalies with the Nd:YAG laser (1.06 μm)[a]

Power	50 W
Spot size	1.5 mm
Pulse duration	cw
Remarks	Cooling of the surface is necessary, water or chlorethyl is not enough. Cooling procedure: ice cubes without air pockets, good skin contact with the ice cube, otherwise burns are possible

[a] Treatment induces vasculitis with subsequent vessel occlusion of the deeper parts

Table 9. Treatment of ectatic veins: percutaneous intraluminal irradiation with the bare fibre, Nd:YAG laser (1.06 μm)[a]

Power	10–20 W
Pulse duration	1–5 s
Speed of withdrawal	0.2–1 mm/s
Remarks	Fibre tip always in saline solution

[a] After puncture of the ectatic veins it is possible to irradiate intraluminally with subsequent shrinkage and occlusion

the resection of angiomas. A focusing handpiece with a focus of 0.5 mm and an output of about 50 W facilitates separation of cavernous haemangiomas and lymphangiomas from the surrounding soft tissue. In order to avoid thermal damage with subsequent uncontrollable coagulation, pulse duration must not exceed 0.3–0.5 s. If necessary it may be helpful to spread the tissue apart with an instrument so that larger vessels can be coagulated with the defocused beam and cut after ligature. Furthermore, the method combines radical resection with protection of functionally important structures. Thus, the residues of angiomas can be coagulated homogeneously with the defocused beam and the formation of secondaries is greatly reduced. Nevertheless, all angiomas on the face and at functionally important sites should be treated promptly; despite the tendency to spontaneous remission their growth can lead to enormous problems in children.

Endoscopy

Diseases of children are very different from those of adults (Table 10). In adults we mostly encounter tumours; in children there are also congenital malformations and traumatic disease [3]. This wide spectrum of diseases encourages the use of a variety of different laser systems, especially the Nd:YAG laser because its radiation can be easily transmitted by fibres (Table 11).

This laser is an ideal instrument for bloodless operations and for tumour destruction. For fine microsurgical work it was formerly regarded as unsuitable. This was the domain of the CO_2 laser even though it was impossible to transmit its radi-

Table 10. Areas of paediatric endoscopy in which lasers facilitate endoscopic surgical procedures

Laryngotracheobronchoscopy
Oesophagogastroduodenoscopy
Procto-recto-coloscopy
Urethro-cystoscopy
Laparoscopy
Thoracoscopy

Table 11. Paediatric endoscopic laser surgery procedures with high success rates

Atresia
Stenosis
Diverticulum
Fistula
Mucosal ectopia
Mucosal hyperplasia
Polyps
Vessel anomalies
Ligaments
Adhesions
Cysts

Table 12. Shrinkage of fistulae and diverticula by contact Nd: YAG laser (1.06 μm), bare fibre, sapphire contact tips[a]

Power	10 W
Pulse duration	1–2 s per area
Speed of withdrawal	0.5–1 mm/s
Remarks	Retrograde procedure only, if necessary use fibrin glue

[a] In paediatric surgery we cannot use sapphire contact tips. In these cases we use the bare fibre and saline solution for shrinkage of fistulae and diverticula

ation by fibres and there was no practical flushing system. An essential advance was the development of sapphire contact tips. Owing to the high energy densities at the needle point and the special beam geometry, very exact work (formation of a coagulation zone about 1.5–2 mm) is possible. This instrumentation can be used for surgery of the outer genitals if an accurate laser application is needed, e.g. for recanalization of hymenal and vaginal atresia or surgery of cloacal malformations. Another application of sapphire contact tips is removal of the remains of recto-urethral or rectovestibular fistulas. With cylindrical or hemispherical sapphire tips the fistula mucosa can be denaturated by laser radiation with an output about 10 W cw, slowly pulling the fibre through the fistula with subsequent shrinkage of the perifistular tissue. In this way risky repeat operations can be avoided (Table 12).

Sometimes sapphire tips cannot be used for endoscopy in children, because they are too large for the infant endoscope. However, with short exposure times of 0.2–0.5 s one can work with the bare fibre without destroying it. This is very helpful for the treatment of diverticula (with subsequent shrinkage) and also for the elimination of urethral valves.

For congenital or scarry stenoses incision and recanalization with even shorter exposure times of 0.1–0.2 s and an output of about 30 W in the contact method with the bare fibre avoid transmural necrosis of tissue and destruction of the organ wall (Tables 13 and 14). It appears that complete removal of the tissue is not always necessary, but that resection of the developing coagulation necrosis finally produces a sufficiently large lumen (Figs. 8 and 9).

Table 13. Treatment of congenital and benign malformations by contact Nd:YAG laser (1.06 μm), bare fibre, sapphire contact tip

Coagulation	
Power	10 W
Pulse duration	0.2–0.5 s
Incision	
Power	15–35 W
Pulse duration	0.2–0.3 s
Remarks	Take care to avoid overheating and coagulation necrosis

Table 14. Treatment of congenital and benign malformations by non-contact Nd:YAG laser (1.06 μm), bare fibre

Coagulation[a]	
Power	15–25 W
Spot size	1.5 mm
Pulse duration	0.2–0.5 s
Incision	
Power	40 W
Spot size	1.5 mm
Pulse duration	0.1 s
Remarks	Take care to avoid overheating and coagulation necrosis

[a] Sometimes it is not necessary to remove all the tissue owing its spontaneous absorption

8 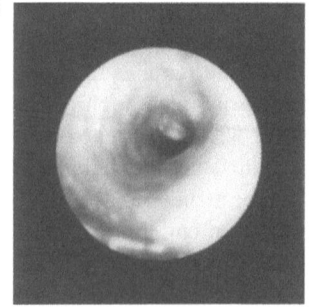 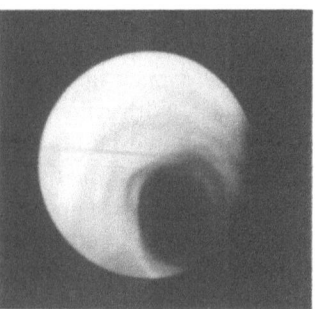 9

Fig. 8. Long-distance trachea stenosis after rib implantation. There is a rest stenosis and granuloma

Fig. 9. After laser coagulation of the granuloma complete healing and epithelialization of the trachea. Complete removal of the granuloma is not necessary. In these cases coagulation with spontaneous resorption is sufficient

Resection

In resection of parenchymatous organs and very bloody tumours, e.g. sarcomas and embryonal tumours, there is always the risk of a large loss of blood (Table 15). In adults this may be tolerable, but for children and especially babies it represents a vital risk. The loss of 50–100 ml of blood by an infant can lead to a state of shock. Therefore, the search for a bloodless anaemic resection method is very important for paediatric surgery. Nevertheless, there remains the problem of radical resection, especially for sarcomas and embryonal tumours. As these tumours often invade the surrounding soft tissue, radical resection can only be achieved with enormous loss of function. For resection of parenchymatous organs and bloody, invasive tumours the Nd:YAG laser has proved very useful [3].

In the past the ultrasound aspirator (CUSA) has been successfully used for liver surgery in adults. With this method one can cut the parenchyma; and all the vessels are saved and can be ligated. Owing to intraoperative bleeding the operation is often carried out by clamping the liver vessels. The subsequent repair of the resection area requires fibrin glue, with the risk of a bleeding beneath the glue layer. Another possibility is the infrared coagulator, but owing to the wavelength of the light the penetration depth in tissue is limited. The CUSA is not suitable for resection of other parenchymatous organs such as lung, spleen, kidney and pancreas. The same applies to the resection of bloody tumours except in neurosurgery.

In the past the Nd:YAG laser was used enthusiastically for liver resection, but success was not always assured. Some people believe there is no place for the Nd:YAG laser in the resection of parenchymatous organs. In experimental research on segmental liver transplantation the procedures for laser resection of parenchymatous organs and bloody tumours should be further developed and standardized.

In order to achieve deep penetration by a sufficiently high power density, with consequent carbonization and vaporization of the tissue, it is necessary to use a focusing handpiece to give a maximum focus of 0.5 mm diameter and minimum

Table 15. Laser resection of parenchymatous organs and tumours

Lung
Liver
Spleen
Pancreas
Kidney
Tumours
    Soft tissue sarcomas
    Intrathoracic neuroblastomas
    Intra-abdominal neuroblastomas
    Teratomas
    Invasive tumours

output at the end of the fibre of 100 W. At lower power density point carbonization and vaporization, necessary for clean cutting, are hard to achieve. The cutting speed must not exceed 1 mm/s, otherwise carbonization will cease owing to cooling of the tissue below 300°C. This procedure allows one to cut the parenchyma without too much loss of blood because veins 3–5 mm in diameter and arteries up to 1.5 mm will be closed primarily. Bigger vessels which have been cut accidently may close up and later supply will be very difficult. It is helpful to compress the resection margin bidigitally and to spread it apart in order to identify bigger vessels in time. The different structure of the vessels compared with the parenchyma allows them to resist the laser beam longer. Therefore they are easy to identify and can be ligated in advance (Table 16).

Especially in resection of the liver and spleen a seeping haemorrhage from the parenchyma can easily be avoided by bidigital compression of the resection margin without clamping off the liver vessels and throttling them. Extravasating blood, which would completely absorb the radiation and hinder the cutting of the tissue, can be eliminated with saline solution under a powerful beam. In this case an infusion pressure system is attached by a small luminous cannula (20 g; Fig. 10), in order to obtain high pressure with a small perfusion volume. Rinsing must occur only intermittently, because continuous rinsing would prevent the carbonization required for tissue cutting. This procedure is especially helpful for spleen and kidney resection (Fig. 11).

This experience has made it possible to carry out resections at the liver, spleen, kidneys and lung successfully, even under difficult conditions. Especially for resections of intrapulmonary metastases it has been found that a bloodless and hermetically sealed resection field develops, so that the danger of hydrothorax and pneumothorax can be reduced, even without additional sutures; it is only necessary to supply the instilled bronchus. Even for extirpation of infiltrated malignant tumours in the abdomen and thorax, sufficiently radical resection with protection of important structures can be performed. The operation takes place at the border of the healthy tissue with an output of 50–60 W, a focus of 0.5 mm and pulses of 0.2–0.3 s duration. If the tissue is slightly spread apart during irradiation, it is possible to operate on the tissue carefully and bloodlessly without uncontrolled tissue necrosis. Larger vessels can either be defocused of coagulated or they can be cut after ligature (Table 17). When a radical resection is not possible, one can homogeneously denature tumour rests at the bottom of the wound by a defocused beam

Table 16. Resection of tumours and parenchymatous organs by the Nd:YAG laser (1.06 μm)

Power	100–120 W
Spot size (by focusing handpiece)	0.5 mm
Pulse duration	cw
Speed	1 mm/s
Remarks	Continous aspiration and intermittent rinsing with high pressure saline solution during resection

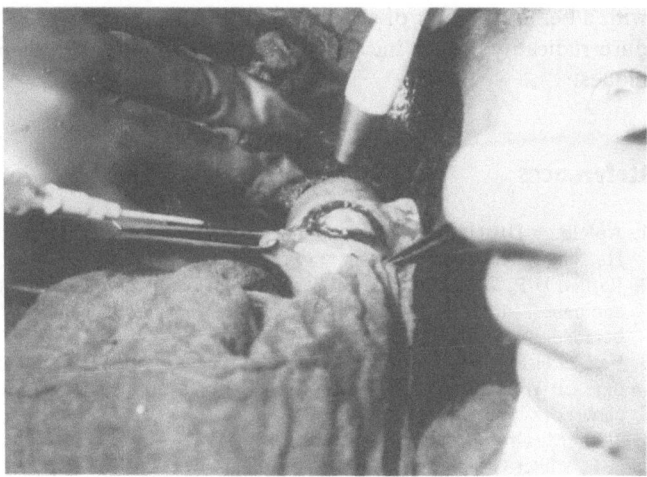

Fig. 10. During organ resection intermittent rinsing with saline solution is successful for removing blood

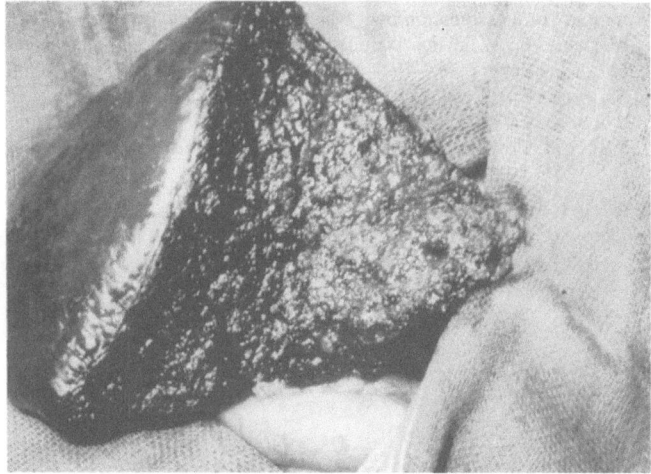

Fig. 11. Hemisplenectomy in Banti's disease. Dry resection surface, fibrin glue and sutures are unnecessary; only ligature of the central vessel is required

Table 17. Separation and resection of tumour tissue by the Nd:YAG laser (1.06 μm)

Power	50 W
Spot size	0.5 mm
Pulse duration	0.2–0.3 s
Remarks	Spreading of tissue, defocused coagulation of bigger vessels, or ligature

with a beam diameter of about 2 mm and an output of 40–50 W. With this procedure radicality can be increased with improvement of functional resection techniques.

References

1. Apfelberg DB (1987) Evaluation and installation of surgical laser systems. Springer, Berlin Heidelberg New York
2. Berlien H-P, Waldschmidt J, Müller G (1988) Laser treatment of cutaneous and deep vessel anomalies. In: Waidelich W (ed) Laser: optoelectronics in medicine. Springer, Berlin Heidelberg New York, pp 526–528
3. Berlien H-P, Biewald W, Waldschmidt J, Müller G (1988) Laser application in pediatric urology. In: Waidelich W (ed) Laser: optoelectronics in medicine. Springer, Berlin Heidelberg New York, pp 341–344
4. Böhm M, Grothues-Spork M, Berlien H-P (1989) Anwendungsfelder des Lasers. In: Berlien H-P, Müller G (eds) Angewandte Lasermedizin, Lehr- und Handbuch für Praxis und Klinik. ecomed, Landsberg
5. Dinstl K, Fischer PL (1981) Der Laser, Grundlagen und klinische Anwendung. Springer, Berlin Heidelberg New York
6. McKenzie AL (1983) How far does thermal damage extend beneath the surface of CO_2 laser incisions? Phys Med Biol 28 (9): 905–912
7. Müller G, Berlien H-P, Biamino G, Dörschel K, Kar H (1988) Photoablation threshold of human aorta as function of wavelength. In: Waidelich W (ed) Laser and optoelectronics in medicine. In: Waidelich W (ed) Laser: optoelectronics in medicine. Springer, Berlin Heidelberg New York, pp 38–41
8. Shriniwasan R, Leigh WT (1986) Ablation of polymers and biological tissue by ultraviolet lasers. Science 234: 559–565
9. Weber H, Herziger G (1984) Lasergrundlagen und -anwendungen. Physik, Weinheim

The Neodymium YAG Laser in Surgery of Parenchymatous Organs in Childhood

P. P. Schmittenbecher

Summary

In seven patients laser resections of liver, spleen and kidney were carried out. Three liver tumours, a hemisplenectomy in Hodgkin's disease, a traumatic spleen injury, an *Echinococcus* infection of the liver and a pole resection in double kidney were dealt with. Healing was undisturbed in all cases, no biliary or urinary fistulae were observed. Further indications are seen in pancreatic and pulmonary resection.

The neodymium YAG laser is a useful instrument in parenchymatous surgery in childhood. Resections are possible without loss of blood and without or with a reduced necessity of transfusion. After traumatic lesions preservation of organs is possible.

Zusammenfassung

Bei 7 Patienten wurden Laserresektionen der Leber, der Milz und der Niere durchgeführt. Es handelte sich um 3 Lebertumoren, eine Hemisplenektomie bei M. Hodgkin, eine traumatische Milzverletzung, eine Echinokokkuserkrankung der Leber und eine Polresektion bei Doppelniere. Die Heilung war in allen Fällen ungestört, es bildeten sich keine Galle- oder Urinfisteln. Weitere Indikationen stellen Pankreas- oder Lungenresektionen dar.

Der Neodym-YAG-Laser ist ein hilfreiches Instrument in der Parenchymchirurgie des Kindesalters. Resektionen können ohne großen Blutverlust und somit ohne oder mit geringeren Fremdblutübertragungen durchgeführt werden. Nach traumatischen Organverletzungen ist ein organerhaltendes Vorgehen möglich.

Résumé

Nous avons partiqué sur 7 patients des résections hépatiques, spléniques et rénales par la méthode du laser. Il s'agissait dans 3 cas de tumeurs du foie, d'une hémisplénectomie au décours d'un Hodgkins, d'un traumatisme de la rate, d'une échinococcose hépatique et d'une résection d'un pôle sur un double rein. Les suites opératoires ont été simples dans tous les cas: pas de fistule, tant au niveau vésiculaire qu'au niveau vésical. La méthode peut être élargie à d'autres indications, par exemple pancréatiques ou pulmonaires.

Le laser Neodym − YAG constitue un instrument de référence dans la chirurgie du parenchyme.

Il permet d'obtenir des sections non hémorragiques et évite ainsi des transfusions sanguines. Il a un effet conservateur lors du traitement chirurgical d'un organe blessé.

Pediatric Surgical Clinic, Dr. von Hauners Childrens Hospital, University of Munich, Lindwurmstrasse 4, D-8000 Munich 2, Federal Republic of Germany

Progress in Pediatric Surgery, Vol. 25
Angerpointner (Ed.)
© Springer-Verlag Berlin Heidelberg 1990

Introduction

In conventional partial resection of parenchymatous organs significant bleeding is one of the main problems, especially in neonates and infants. The patients rapidly lose considerable amounts of their small blood volume. Laser light leads to photo-thermal effects in tissue and causes coagulation, drying up, carbonization and evaporization, depending on the temperature.

The neodymium YAG laser emits nonvisible light in the near infrared with a wavelength of 1.06 μm. This wavelength implies a relatively deep penetration into the tissue. This laser system, properly a coagulation laser, achieves its cutting effect by its high power density [9]. Because of thermal radiation in all directions, both sides of the section plane are coagulated as a positive side effect. Thus, in parenchymatous organs a combination of resection and sealing of the cut vessels and ducts, up to a limited diameter, is obtained.

Laser Instruments

We use a neodymium-YAG laser mediLas 2 (MBB-Medizintechnik, D-8012 Ottobrunn, Federal Republic of Germany), wavelength 1.06 μm, maximal power output around 110 W (Fig. 1). Normally we prefer to work without tissue contact,

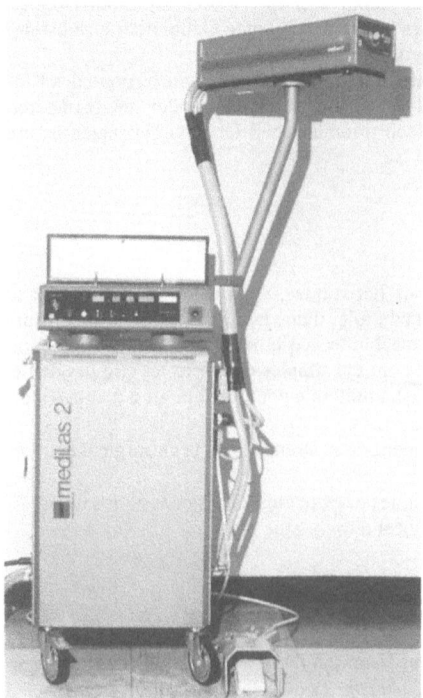

Fig. 1. The Nd-YAG laser system mediLas 2 with maximal power output around 100 W

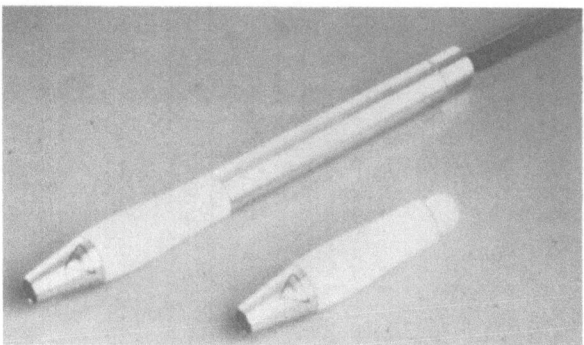

Fig. 2. The focusing handpiece with focal distance of 50 mm

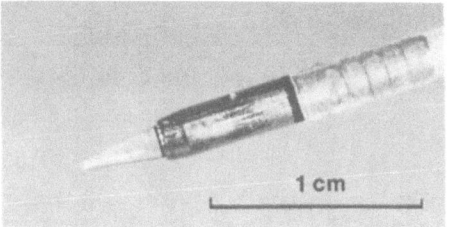

Fig. 3. The sapphire tip, useful in difficult preparations

using the focusing handpiece to focus the laser beam 50 mm in front of the optical system (Fig. 2). It is advantageous to work with tissue contact using a sapphire tip with a small laser beam diameter in difficult preparations (Fig. 3).

Operation Mode

In organ resection full power is necessary. The laser beam should have 100 W power output at the tip of the optical fibre for efficient cutting of tissue. Lower output yields unsatisfactory results. If the sapphire tip is used 25 W is the maximum energy output, since higher energy destroys the sapphire. For exact adjustment of laser power in this lower range it is helpful to have a mode diaphragm fixed in the laser which allows one to fine tune the energy between 0 and 30 W.

In both modes of operation, spreading of the initial tissue incision allows optimal positioning of the laser beam and early recognition of larger vessels (diameter ≥ 5 mm) for ligation. Intermittent irrigation prevents loss of energy due to absorption by blood.

Clinical Applications

Case 1. A 20-month-old girl presented with an abdominal mass. A CT scan and an angiogram showed a large tumour of the right and middle lobe of the liver. Resec-

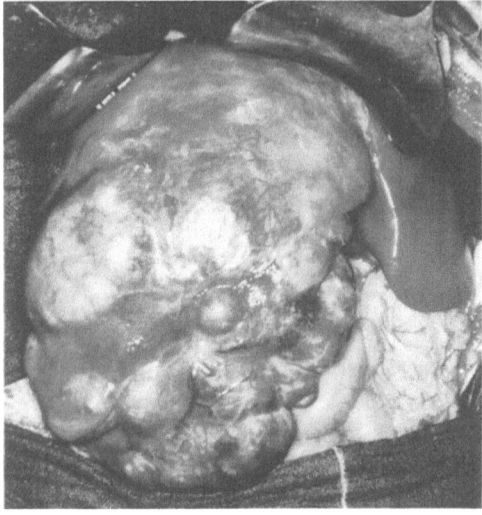

Fig. 4. Patient 1. Large nodose tumour in the right and middle lobe of the liver

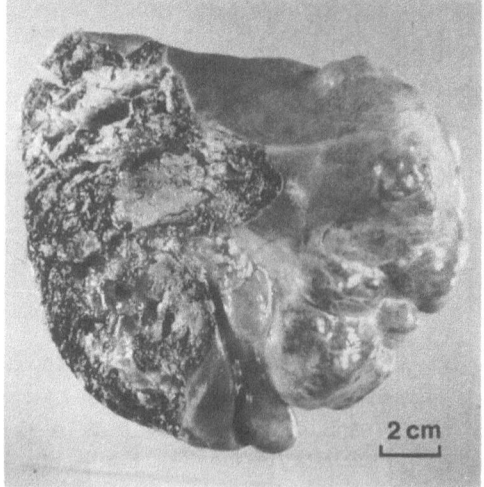

2 cm

Fig. 5. The resected liver tumour with dry resection plane

tion was performed with the neodymium-YAG laser after clamping and ligation of large vessels (Figs. 4 and 5). We used the focusing handpiece and the full power of the laser (100 W). Resection time was 50 min without further need of haemostasis. Neither intraoperatively nor postoperatively was blood transfusion necessary. Pathohistological examination revealed a hepatoblastoma without infiltration of surrounding structures.

Case 2. A 13-year-old boy with erythroleukaemia in full remission developed an intrahepatic granuloma following *Candida* infection (Fig. 6). Surgical removal was

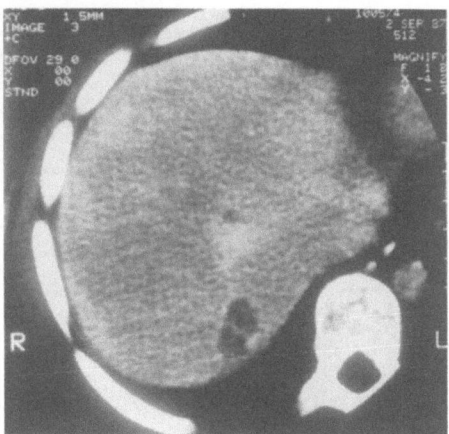

Fig. 6. Patient 2. Hepatic granuloma in the posterior part of the liver visualized on a CT scan

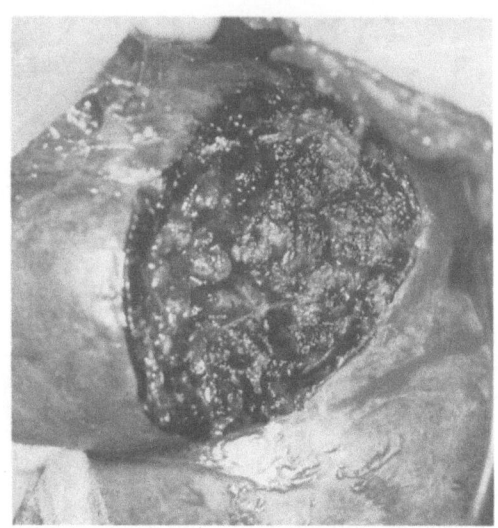

Fig. 7. The area of the granuloma after excision without bleeding

necessary prior to autologous bone marrow transplantation. The dorsally located granuloma was excised with the focusing handpiece and high power without further preparation of the vessels (Fig. 7). No blood transfusion was necessary and the postoperative course was without complications.

Case 3. A 12-year-old boy from Yugoslavia was transferred to our hospital for suspected *Echinococcus* infection. Ultrasound examination showed seven intrahepatic cysts all round the liver (Fig. 8). These cystic structures and their capsules were marsupialized (Fig. 9). We used the sapphire tip and energy output between 15 and 20 W, incised the tissue above the cysts and removed them by laser and blunt

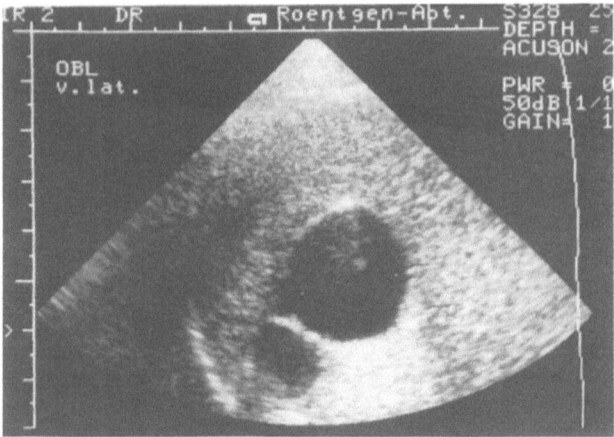

Fig. 8. Patient 3. Typical ultrasonic finding in *Echinococcus* cysts with septa

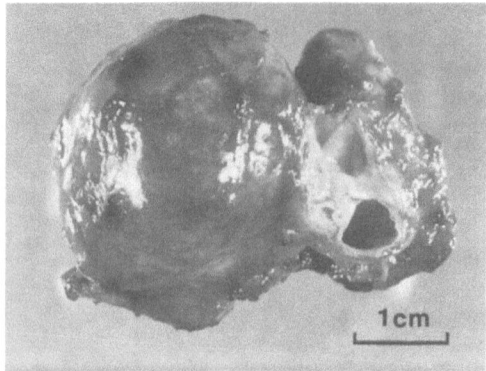

Fig. 9. The largest of seven *Echinococcus* cysts excised

dissection. Intraoperative ultrasonic control was very helpful. No blood transfusion was necessary and no problems in wound healing were observed. Histologically *Echinococcus cysticus* was found.

Case 4. An 11-year-old boy with Hodgkin's disease needed to undergo staging laparotomy. Hemisplenectomy was carried out with the laser and focusing handpiece (Figs. 10 and 11).

Case 5. A 15-year-old boy had undergone radiotherapy and chemotherapy for Ewing's sarcoma. CT scan carried out for exclusion of pulmonary metastasis disclosed a previously unknown tumour of the left lobe of the liver. Intraoperatively, this turned out to be a solid process (6 cm diameter) at the ventral edge of the left lobe of the liver (Fig. 12) which was easily excised by laser. Histological exami-

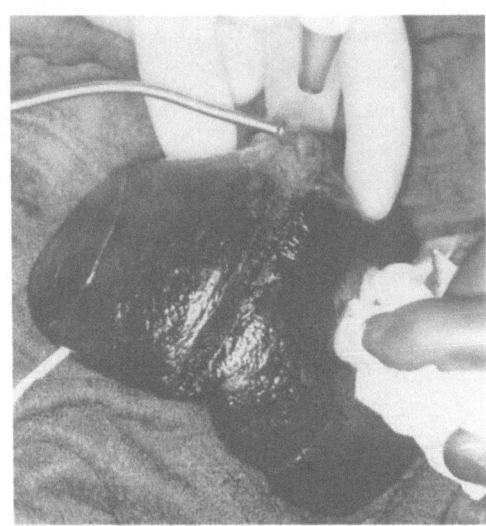

Fig. 10. Patient 4. During hemi-splenectomy. The incision groove is spread apart by the operating surgeon, the smoke is removed by suction

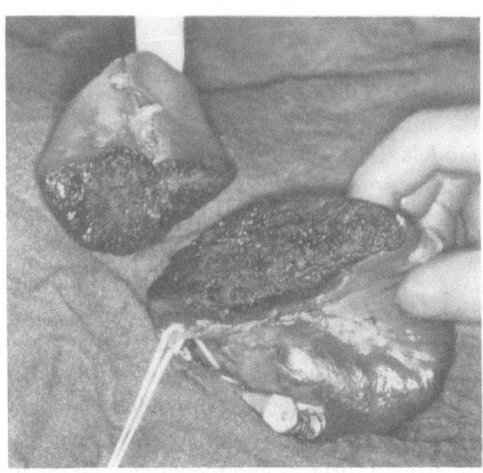

Fig. 11. After separation of the two parts of the spleen. The section plane remains dry

nation demonstrated a benign hepatoma, supposedly a consequence of former chemotherapy. Preoperatively haemoglobin was 13.2 mg%, postoperatively 12.5 mg%.

Case 6 and 7. In a patient with a double kidney the upper pole was resected by laser without bleeding from the resection plane. Another girl was transferred to our hospital for after-bleeding following a kick from a horse; she also had an outside hemisplenectomy. The diffuse bleeding from the resection area was stopped by superficial laser coagulation with a defocused beam and energy of 40 W.

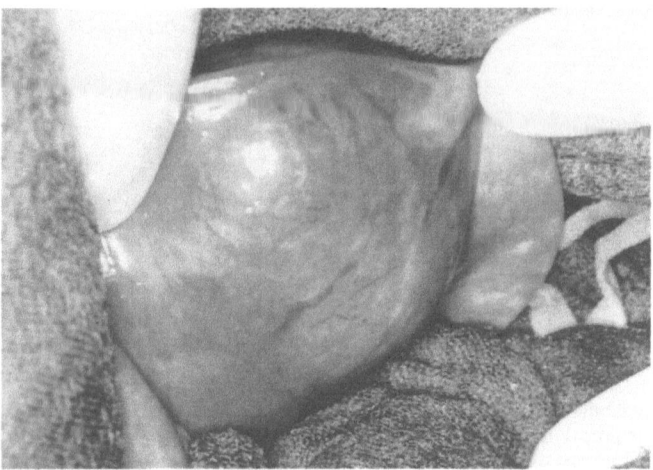

Fig. 12. Patient 5. Hepatoma at the ventral edge of the left lobe of the liver

Discussion

Laser techniques have been applied in surgery of parenchymatous organs since the middle of the 1970s after the prerequisites had been established in animal models. Bödecker et al. [2] and Grotelüschen et al. [5] first described the energy distribution and the morphological tissue alterations after Nd YAG laser application. In 1980 Karbe et al. [6] investigated the applicability of the Neodymium-YAG laser for liver resection in pigs and for kidney pole resection in dogs. The resection itself took longer than in alternative methods, but, in contrast to the CO_2 laser or the electric knife, the Neodymium-YAG laser yielded a bloodless resection surface owing to coagulation and vessel thrombosis. The healing of the resection wound in parenchymatous tissue was not impaired by the carbonization of the surface. Having performed liver resections in pigs without preparation of the vessels, Meyer and Haverkamp [8] gave the typical coagulation depth as 5 mm at the wound surfaces and recommended the neodymium YAG laser as a good combination of cutting and coagulation. They stressed the possibility of stopping minor bleeding by use of the defocused laser beam. Godlewski et al. [4] first used a commercial neodymium-YAG laser system for liver resection in pigs. The largest diameter of vessels securely sealed by the laser was 4.5 mm. Furthermore, Meier et al. [7] showed the formation of a neocapsule after laser resection in rabbit liver, spleen and kidney over a period of 2–3 weeks. No fistulae from bile ducts or the urinary system could be demonstrated by any group.

The somewhat wider incision groove and a transitory increase of liver enzymes are the only drawbacks, while the advantages are bloodless resection, no afterbleeding, formation of a neocapsule and the absence of fistulae or healing disturbances. Therefore the laser technique has been introduced into clinical practice.

Table 1. Indications for laser surgery in parenchymatous organs

Liver	Tumour, rupture, solitary metastasis, resection for transplantation, resection in inflammatory disease or error of metabolism
Spleen	Rupture, resection for staging of Hodgkin's disease
Kidney	Pole resection in double kidney, tumour in single kidney or in both kidneys
Pancreas	Tumour, rupture, pseudocyst
Lung	Metastasis

The largest clinical experience with lasers in paediatric surgery is reported by Berlien [1]. Further indications are mentioned by Meier et al. [7]. Table 1 lists the indications for laser surgery of parenchymatous organs in children as described in the literature.

No published clinical case has ever reported a fistula from bile duct, urinary system, bronchus or pancreatic duct. The somewhat longer duration of the resection procedure is compensated because no further haemostasis is necessary. The total operation time is the same or even shorter.

In adult surgery laser systems are seldom used for resection of parenchymatous organs [10]. The greater diameter of vessels in adult organs may impair the optimal haemostasis as observed in experiments and in paediatric surgical use. However, in segmental lung resections DeCaro [3] showed successful laser application with alveolar sealing and without persistent air leaks.

The Neodymium-YAG laser system extends the technical possibilities of surgery in parenchymatous organs. The aim of organ preservation, especially in childhood, will be greatly enhanced by laser techniques. Laser surgery is also of advantage in reducing the need for blood transfusions.

References

1. Berlien H-P (1987) Therapeutische Leitlinien zur Laserbehandlung. LMZ, Berlin
2. Bödecker V, Rudolph M, Grotelüschen B (1974) Messung der Intensitätsverteilung von YAG-Laserstrahlung im Gewebe. Biomed Technol 19:160–162
3. DeCaro LF (1987) Nd-YAG laser segmental resection for lung cancer. Tumor Diagn Ther 7 [Suppl]:47–49
4. Godlewski G, Ginoves P, Chincholles JM, Viel E, Bureau JP, Rouy S, Mion H, Dubois A, Fesquet J (1983) Hepatic resection with an Nd-YAG laser in pig. Lasers Surg Med 3:217–224
5. Grotelüschen B, Rauner P, Bödecker V, Sepold G (1974) Morphologische Befunde bei Schnittversuchen an der Rattenleber mittels Neodymlaser. Biomed Technol 19:75–78
6. Karbe E, Königsmann G, Beck R (1980) Experimentelle Leber- und Nierenchirurgie mit dem CO_2-, CO-, Holmium- und Neodym-Laser. Langenbecks Arch Chir 351:179–192
7. Meier H, Dietl KH, Stöhr G, Willital GH (1986) Experience of neodym-YAG-laser in pediatric surgery. Laser 2:68–74
8. Meyer H-J, Haverkamp K (1982) Experimental study of partial liver resection with a combined CO_2 and Nd-YAG laser. Lasers Surg Med 2:149–154
9. Müller G, Berlien H-P, Scholz G (1986) Laser in medicine. Laser 2:78–87
10. Wacha H (1987) Laser-Chirurgie: Vorzüge, Grenzen. Dtsch Arztebl 84:3532–3536

Haemostasis in Injuries of Parenchymatous Organs by Infrared Contact Coagulation

T. A. Angerpointner[1], K. L. Lauterjung[2], and A. Hoffecker[1]

Summary

A series of 11 children aged from 1 day to 12 years is reported in which infrared contact coagulation with a sapphire coagulator was used for haemostasis in liver and splenic injuries. Seven children were cured. The four deaths were not related to the injuries of parenchymatous organs. Infrared contact coagulation is a suitable and cheap method for organ preservation in injuries or other pathological conditions of parenchymatous organs in childhood.

Zusammenfassung

Es wird über eine Serie von 11 Kindern im Alter von 1 Tag bis 12 Jahren berichtet, bei denen die Infrarotkontaktkoagulation mit einem Saphirkoagulator zur Blutstillung bei Leber- und Milzverletzungen zum Einsatz kam. 7 Kinder wurden als geheilt entlassen. Die 4 Todesfälle standen in keinem Zusammenhang mit den Verletzungen der parenchymatösen Organe. Die Infrarotkontaktkoagulation ist eine geeignete und billige Methode zur Organerhaltung bei Verletzungen oder anderen pathologischen Zuständen parenchymatöser Organe im Kindesalter.

Résumé

Sur une série de 11 enfants âgés de 1 à 12 ans a été essayé un coagulateur à infrarouges pour infiltration hémorragique au niveau du foie et de la rate. 7 enfants ont été guéris par cette méthode. Les 4 cas mortels étaient sans rapport avec le traumatisme de l'organe. Cette méthode de coagulation par infrarouges est à la fois parfaitement adaptée et peu onéreuse soit pour la conservation d'organes blessés, soit dans le traitement de tout parenchyme pathologique.

Introduction

Diffuse haemorrhage caused by liver and splenic injuries is sometimes difficult to control. Therefore splenectomy or extended liver operations were often the treatment of choice in the past. However, the first aim in the treatment of injured parenchymatous organs in children is organ preservation, above all preservation of the spleen. Immunological competence of the spleen (one-quarter of the body's

---

[1]Paediatric Surgical Clinic, Dr. von Hauners Childrens Hospital, University of Munich, Lindwurmstrasse 4, D-8000 München 2, Federal Republic of Germany
[2]University Surgical Hospital Munich − Klinikum Großhadern, Marchioninistrasse 15, D-8000 München 70, Federal Republic of Germany

Progress in Pediatric Surgery, Vol. 25
Angerpointner (Ed.)
© Springer-Verlag Berlin Heidelberg 1990

lymphatic tissue) [2] was fully recognized only recently [6]. Great efforts were therefore made to preserve parenchymatous organs after injuries such as abdominal blunt trauma or other pathological conditions such as congenital splenic cyst or common liver in conjoined twins [3]. Preservation of the spleen is of particular importance in preventing overwhelming postsplenectomy sepsis due to impaired immunological function [2, 9]. Infrared contact coagulation of parenchymatous organs in adult patients was described by Lauterjung et al. [7, 8]. So far, we have applied this method in 11 children, achieving complete haemostasis of liver and splenic haemorrhage.

Patients and Method

The method of infrared contact coagulation was developed by Guthy et al. [4]. Höllerl et al. [5] and Lauterjung et al. [7, 8] reported on clinical experience in adult patients. We used the ISK 250 sapphire coagulator (NK-Optik, Forstenrieder Allee 223b, D-8000 München 71, Federal Republic of Germany; Fig. 1).

By means of absorption by the bleeding tissue, light is converted into thermal energy, thus causing coagulation and haemostasis. The light is transmitted to the bleeding tissue via a sapphire crystal which is nonadhesive and of high thermal resistance (melting point 2050°C). Coagulation heads of different geometry (Fig. 1) allow haemostasis on plane surfaces and in fissured tissue where access is difficult.

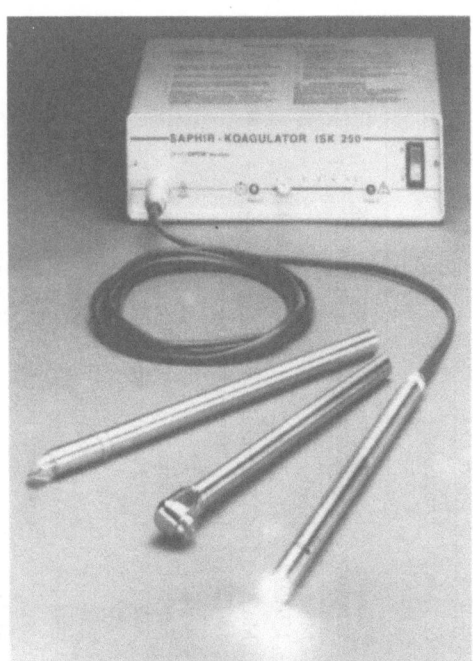

Fig. 1. The ISK 250 infrared sapphire coagulator

Table 1. Infrared contact coagulation in 11 patients: indications and outcome

Patient, sex, date of birth	Diagnosis	Age at operation	Treatment	Outcome
1. Female, 16/3/1970	Delayed splenic rupture following abdominal blunt trauma	12 years	Infrared coagulation of multiple splenic tears	Cured
2. Male, 1/1/1972	Epithelial cyst of the spleen	10 years	Cyst excision and infrared coagulation of diffuse haemorrhage	Cured
3. Male, 18/12/1978	Abdominothoracopagus with common liver (among other anomalies)	3 years	Separation of conjoined twins, infrared coagulation of separated liver surfaces	Twin I cured, twin II died 3 months postoperatively of incurable bowel obstruction
4. Female, 22/2/1984	Abdominopagus with common liver (among other anomalies)	1 day	Emergency separation of conjoined twins, infrared coagulation of separated liver surfaces	Twin I cured, twin II died immediately postoperatively of severe multiple malformations
5. Female, 23/4/1986	Twins, premature birth, necrotizing enterocolitis with bowel perforation, iatrogenic liver tear	2 weeks	Ileostomy, infrared coagulation of liver tear	Died 10 days postoperatively of sepsis and renal insufficiency
6. Male, 7/12/1985	Traffic accident, splenic rupture	2 years	Infrared coagulation of splenic rupture	Cured
7. Male, 29/4/1985	Traffic accident, polytrauma, splenic rupture	2 years	Infrared coagulation of splenic rupture	Cured
8. Male, 4/6/1987	Meconium peritonitis, small bowel atresia, biliary atresia, mucoviscidosis, iatrogenic liver tear intraoperatively	1 day	Ileostomy, infrared coagulation of liver tear	Died 3 months postoperatively of underlying disease
9. Female, 13/2/1981	Kicked by a horse, liver rupture	6 years	Infrared coagulation of liver rupture	Cured
10. Female, 21/8/1976	Fall from trampoline, splenic rupture	12 years	Infrared coagulation of splenic rupture	Cured
11. Female, 14/4/1988	Necrotizing enterocolitis, perforation of the left colonic flexure, iatrogenic splenic tear intraoperatively	3 days	Colostomy, infrared coagulation of splenic tear	Cured

An automatic device, which adjusts coagulation time up to 5 s continuously, provides individual adaptation to different organ sizes and thus application of the method in neonates.

Diagnosis, age at operation, treatment and outcome in the 11 children are summarized in Table 1. Their ages ranged from 1 day to 12 years. The spleen was affected in 6 cases and the liver in 5 cases. A common liver bridge had to be dissected in two pairs of conjoined twins (cases 3 and 4). Case 3 was described in detail by Grantzow et al. [3]. In the first pair of conjoined twins one twin was

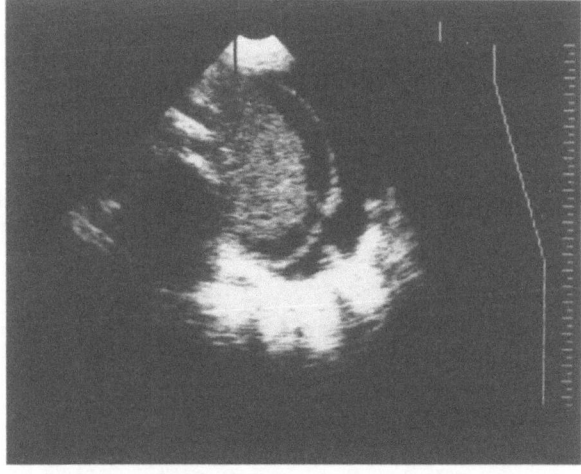

Fig. 2. Abdominal ultrasound revealing a large falciform subcapsular splenic haematoma

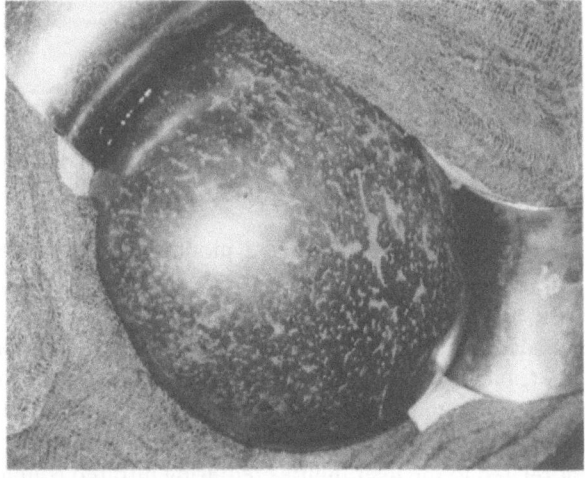

Fig. 3. Protruding spleen after laparotomy. Note enlargement and tension on the splenic capsule

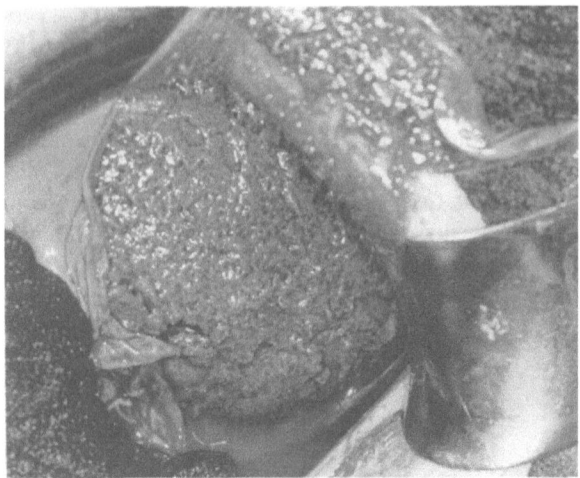

Fig. 4. Splenic tissue following removal of the capsule. Note deep fissure at the lower pole

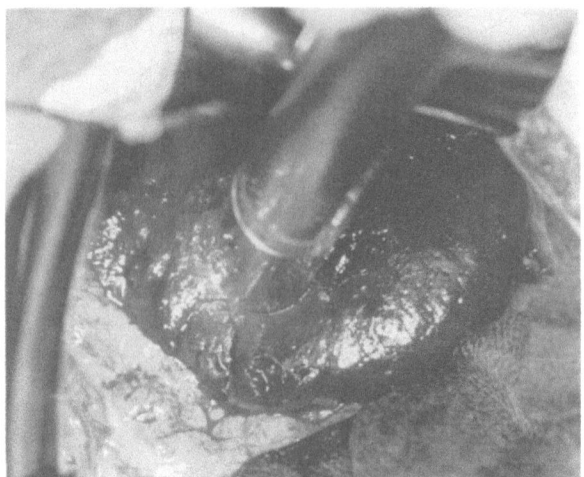

Fig. 5. Infrared coagulation head in situ for coagulation of splenic fissure

cured, whereas the other died 3 months postoperatively of sepsis and incurable bowel obstruction. In the other pair of conjoined twins, who had to be separated at the age of few hours as an emergency, one twin was cured and the other died immediately after surgery of severe multiple malformations such as tetralogy of Fallot, biliary duct aplasia and pancreatic agenesis. The other two deaths in the series were due to postoperative sepsis and renal insufficiency and to the severe underlying disease of the infant (mucoviscidosis, biliary atresia). The deaths were not related to the liver injuries requiring infrared contact coagulation. One case is described in detail.

Case Report: A 12-year-old girl sustained an abdominal blunt trauma while skating in 1981. She did not attend a physician thereafter. During the following 2 months she developed increasing abdominal pain and recurrent vomiting. When she was hospitalized 2 months after the accident, a palpable mass in the upper left abdominal quadrant was found to extend beyond the midline to the right. Chest X-ray showed left-sided diaphragmatic elevation. Abdominal ultrasound (Fig. 2) disclosed a falciform accumulation of fluid between the splenic capsule and the parenchyma. Blood counts and chemistry were normal. On laparotomy (Fig. 3) a large subcapsular haematoma containing approximately 1 l of old blood was found. After resection of the separated splenic capsule (Fig. 4) a deep fissure in the lower splenic pole was found which began to bleed again after removal of the splenic capsule. Complete haemostasis was achieved by means of infrared contact coagulation (Fig. 5) thus providing preservation of the spleen. The postoperative course was entirely uneventful. Postoperative splenic scintiscan showed normal size and pattern.

Comments

Initial experience with infrared contact coagulation in children was reported by us in 1983 [1]. The initial drawbacks of infrared coagulation, such as thermal destruction of the coagulation head, were overcome by the development of a sapphire crystal of high thermal resistance as the transmitter between light source and bleeding tissue [4, 7, 8].

The following requirements are fulfilled by the sapphire coagulator: tissue coagulation to a depth of 5 mm, thus providing secure haemostasis; high energy output for effective coagulation, minimal adhesiveness of the sapphire crystal; coagulation heads of different geometries for application on plane surfaces and in deep fissures where access is difficult; high thermal and chemical resistance; normal sterilization; and low working voltage.

The main benefits of infrared contact coagulation are cheapness, easy handling, very rapid haemostasis in wet tissue, large area of the coagulation head and deep coagulation of parenchymatous tissue up to 5 mm. Infrared contact coagulation is a valuable method for preservation of injured parenchymatous organs in paediatric surgery.

References

1. Angerpointner TA, Lauterjung KL, Holschneider AM, Hecker WC (1983) Infrared contact coagulation of parenchymatous organs − report of three cases. Z Kinderchir 38:356–358
2. Belohradsky BH, Däumling S, Roos R, Holschneider AM, Griscelli C (1982) Postsplenectomy infections and *pneumococcus* vaccination in paediatric surgery. Z Kinderchir 35:140–144
3. Grantzow R, Hecker W, Holschneider AM, Mantel K, Carrier B (1985) Trennung eines asymmetrischen Xipho-Omphalo-Ischiopagus tripus. Langenbecks Arch Chir 363:195–206

4. Guthy E, Kiefhaber P, Nath G, Kreitmayr A (1979) Infrared coagulation. Clinical application in liver and spleen. Langenbecks Arch Chir 348:105–108
5. Höllerl G, Höfler H, Tscheliessnigg KH, Hermann W, Stenzl W, Dacar D (1982) Infrarot-Kontaktkoagulation zur Blutstillung an Leber und Milz. Fortschr Med 100:347–351
6. Holschneider AM, Kricz-Klimeck H, Strasser B, Däumling S, Belohradsky BH (1982) Complications after splenectomy in childhood. Z Kinderchir 35:130–139
7. Lauterjung KL, Nath G, Seifert J, Brandel W, Guthy E (1981) Blutstillung an Leber und Milz mit einem Infrarot-Saphir-Koagulator. Langenbecks Arch Chir 355:646–648
8. Lauterjung KL, Nath G, Heberer G (1982) Blutstillung mit einem neuen Infrarot-Saphir-Coagulator (ISC 81). Chirurg 53:88–92
9. Singer DB, Rosenberg HS, Bolande RP (1973) Perspectives in pediatric pathology. I. Year Book Medical Publishers, Chicago, pp 285–311

The Shaw Haemostatic Scalpel in Paediatric Surgery: Clinical Report on 3000 Operations

U. G. Stauffer

Summary

This report presents the experience in a prospective series of 100 operative procedures in all fields of paediatric surgery with the Shaw haemostatic scalpel, which we have subsequently used in more than 3000 further operations. The Shaw scalpel proved to be advantageous in about 80% of major cases. The scalpel cuts tissue with a sharp steel edge, like a cold scalpel, and simultaneously seals blood vessels by heat thermally conducted to the tissue from heated blade which is electrically insulated from the patient. The heat seals most small blood vessels (under 2 mm) as they are cut. Since no electric current passes through the patient, a grounding pad is not needed and the risk of accidental electrical current burns at grounding sites is eliminated. Muscle stimulation associated with the use of a normal cautery is avoided, improving surgical precision of cutting. The Shaw haemostatic scalpel minimizes damage to the tissue as compared with other thermocoagulating instruments. Since it seals small vessels as it cuts tissue, it largely eliminates the flow of blood into the incised area and allows better visibility of the surgical field. The use of the scalpel requires a different cutting technique which is however easy to learn. The Shaw haemostatic scalpel reduces blood loss and overall operating time in major cases. It is relatively inexpensive and can be recommended for use in paediatric surgery.

Zusammenfassung

Es wird über Erfahrungen bei 100 kinderchirurgischen Operationen auf nahezu allen Gebieten der Kinderchirurgie mit dem Shaw Hemostatic Scalpel berichtet; nach dieser ersten Versuchsserie haben die Autoren das Instrument bis heute in mehr als 3000 weiteren Operationen verwendet. Das Shaw Hemostatic Scalpel erwies sich als günstig in mehr als 80% der größeren Eingriffe. Es schneidet das Gewebe mit einer scharfen Stahlklinge wie ein normales Skalpell und versiegelt gleichzeitig die Blutgefäße durch Hitzekoagulation. Die Klinge wird auf einer gewünschten Temperatur zwischen 110 und 260°C konstant gehalten. Die drei in der Klinge enthaltenen elektrisch geregelten Temperaturelemente sind vom Patienten isoliert. Blutgefäße von 2 mm Durchmesser und weniger werden während des Schneidens verschlossen. Da kein elektrischer Strom durch den Patienten geht, ist eine Erdung nicht nötig, und das Risiko elektrischer Verbrennungen ist ausgeschlossen. Dies ist in Anbetracht der zahlreichen modernen Überwachungsgeräte, die diese Gefahr vergrößern, von besonders großer Bedeutung. Auch kommt es nicht zu Muskelzuckungen, die sich beim Schneiden mit dem üblichen elektrischen Messer ergeben. Das Shaw Hemostatic Scalpel setzt einen geringeren Gewebeschaden als das handelsübliche elektrische Messer. Da die Gefäße bei der Gewebedurchtrennung verschlossen werden, wird das Einströmen von Blut in das Operationsfeld weitgehend vermieden. Dies erlaubt eine "bloodless surgery" mit entsprechend besserer Detailsicht im Operationsfeld. Der Gebrauch dieses Messers erfordert eine etwas andere Schnitttechnik, die jedoch leicht zu erlernen ist. Das Shaw Hemostatic Scalpel reduziert den Blutverlust und die Operationszeit bei größeren chirurgischen Eingriffen. Es ist relativ preisgünstig und kann für den Gebrauch in der Kinderchirurgie empfohlen werden.

Surgical Department, University Children's Hospital, Steinwiesstrasse 75, CH-8032 Zürich, Switzerland

Progress in Pediatric Surgery, Vol. 25
Angerpointner (Ed.)
© Springer-Verlag Berlin Heidelberg 1990

Résumé

Nous rapportons 100 observations de chirurgie infantile pratiquée avec le bistouri hémostatique de Robert Shaw. Par la suite, nous avons pratiqué 3000 autres interventions par cette méthode. Ce système de bistouri hémostatique fut particulièrement bien adapté dans 80% des interventions. La section pratiquée est aussi fine que celle d'un scalpel usuel et s'assortit d'une hémostase immédiate par coagulation. La lame doit être maintenue à une température oscillant entre 110 et 260°C. Les éléments chauffants électriques de la lame sont bien évidemment isolés du patient. Pour les vaisseaux sanguins d'un diamètre égal ou inférieur à 2 mm, une hémostase spontanée a lieu pendant la section même. Une prise de terre n'est pas nécessaire et tout risque de brûlure est écarté du fait qu'aucun courant électrique ne traverse le patient. Ceci est primordial, étant donné la multiplication des appareils de surveillance électriques.

Autre avantage: l'absence de conduction électrique à travers le patient évite toute contraction musculaire, chose que l'on trouve à l'utilisation du bistouri électrique habituel. Les lésions du bistouri Shaw sont moindres que celles provoquées par les bistouris électriques habituels. Cette hémostase spontanée permet d'éviter une déperdition sanguine per-opératoire. De plus, la sécheresse de la plaie permet une meilleure vision du champ opératoire. Si l'utilisation de ce bistouri nécessite une nouvelle technique, celle-ci est particulièrement simple à acquérir.

Cet instrument permet à la fois une réduction des pertes sanguines et du temps opératoire au cours de la chirurgie lourde. Autre avantage: son prix modique.

Introduction

Haemostasis is an important and frequently time-consuming part of surgery. Precise control of bleeding during operative procedures is an essential tool, especially in the paediatric age group. This is a report on our experience with the Shaw haemostatic scalpel in 3000 operations at our paediatric surgical centre. We started testing this system in a prospective series of 100 cases in 1982. By 1987, about 100 surgeons were on the users reference list for the Shaw scalpel in the United States. There are some reports on the successful use of this scalpel in animal experimental surgery and some favourable reports in different fields of surgery in humans [1–10]. However, the Shaw haemostatic scalpel is not well known amongst paediatric surgeons, especially in Europe and there are no reports on its regular use in this field so far. Our positive experience justifies this report.

Description of the System

The haemostatic scalpel or "hot knife" was invented by Robert Shaw, M.D., a cardiovascular surgeon, and is manufactured by Oximetrix Incorporated Mountain View, California, United States (Fig. 1). The Shaw scalpel system consists of three components: an electronic controller instrument; a reusable scalpel handle connected to the controller by a lightweight, flexible electrical cable; and sterile disposable scalpel blades. The controller unit operates on the standard hospital power supply (115 or 120 V, 50–60 Hz) to provide a pulsed direct current used to heat the scalpel to a selected temperature in the range 110°–260°C. The controller provides an audible tone and visual display to show system operating status and

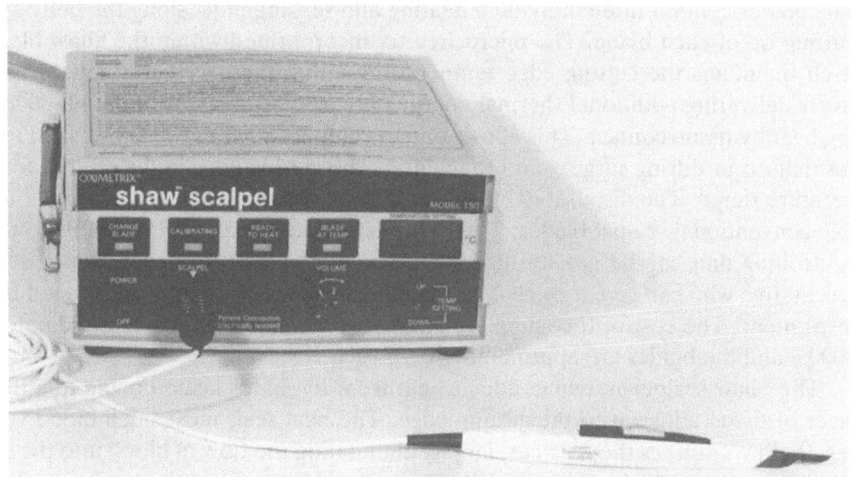

Fig. 1. The Shaw haemostatic scalpel. The controller unit and the handle with the blade

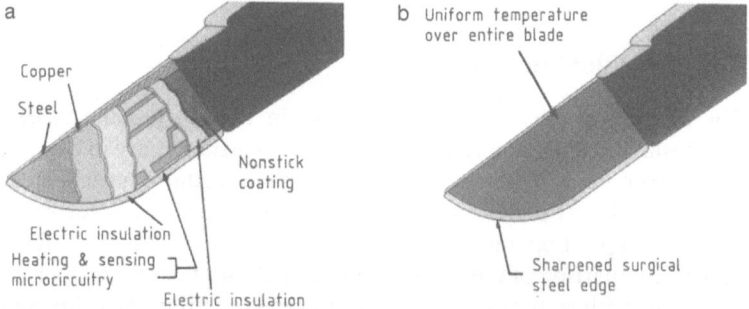

Fig. 2a, b. The Shaw haemostatic blade. **a** "Structure" (see text), **b** Teflon coating

blade temperature setting. The controller senses and powers microelectronic circuitry in the scalpel blade to maintain the blade at the desired temperature within extremely narrow limits. This permits the surgeon to maintain careful control over the degree of thermal injury produced in the tissue. The temperature can be controlled and raised in 10° increments by a small button enclosed in the scalpel handle. When the blade is turned on, it reaches the desired temperature within 3–4 s and when it is turned off, it cools very rapidly. The Shaw blades are individually packed, sterile and ready for use. They are similar in size and shape to conventional scalpel blades (No. 10 and 15) and have the same sharp surgical steel cutting edges to retain the precision and feel of the cold scalpel when cutting. They are constructed from surgical steel and coated with copper and a Teflon (PTEE) outer coating, except for the cutting edge (Fig. 2a, b). The Teflon coating is important since coagulated blood tends to collect on the scalpel. With the Teflon coating, the blade can be easily cleaned by gentle wiping on a sterile gauze.

The blades contain three individual heating and sensing units along the belly and cutting tip of each blade. The microcircuitry incorporated within the Shaw blade itself maintains the cutting edge temperature within the necessary limits, selectively delivering additional thermal energy only to those regions of the blade losing heat by tissue contact. This allows one to compensate for the varying heat losses that occur during surgery and to maintain the cutting edge in the desired temperature range. The disposable blades are discarded when they become dull, just like conventional scalpel blades. The reusable scalpel handle and the cable to the controlling unit can be gas sterilized. The manufacturer provides a trained representative who can give technical instruction on the design and proper use of the instrument. The cost of the complete Shaw haemostatic scalpel is approximately 3000 # and the blades are approximately $ 6 each.

The Shaw scalpel system conducts heat from its sharp, heated blade to a thin layer of tissue adjacent to the cutting edge. The heat seals most small blood vessels (below 2 mm) as they are cut, largely eliminating the flow of blood into the incised area. Since the blade is electrically insulated from the patient, and no electric current passes through the patient, no grounding pad is needed. Muscle stimulation associated with passing electric current through the body is also eliminated.

The First Pilot Study of 100 Cases

The theoretical advantages prompted us in 1982 to test the value of the Shaw haemostatic scalpel in different fields of paediatric surgery in a prospective series of 100 operations. With a few exceptions, all procedures have been carried out by the author. Every patient had a special questionnaire noting temperatures used at different steps of operation, number and quality of blades used during the procedure, a comparison of the haemostatic scalpel with the cold scalpel and electrosurgical units with respect to the amount of time required, the estimated tissue damage, visibility of the operating field and the quantity of fluid administered to the patient. The patients were carefully followed postoperatively for any complications, especially wound healing, infections and cosmetic appearance of the scar at late follow-up.

Results

A total of 90 children with an age range from 1 day to 15 years underwent altogether 100 different procedures which are listed in Table 1.

General Evaluation and Technical Considerations

The effective use of the thermally regulated haemostatic scalpel required development of a different technique from the one we were using before. Surgeons are usually accustomed to cut tissues rapidly and then return to the same area to coagulate bleeding vessels which have been cut. With the Shaw haemostatic scal-

Table 1. Shaw haemostatic scalpel in paediatric surgery: diagnoses in the first 100 pilot cases

Neonatal surgery	
Intestinal malrotation, duodenal atresia, etc.	3
Enterostomy (NEC)	6
Sacroperineal pull-through in anorectal atresia	4
Gastrostomy	4
Abdominal and general surgery	
Hepatoportoenterostomy (Kimura-Kasai)	2
Splenectomy	2
Hemisplenectomy	2
Excision of mesenteric lymph node	4
Appendectomy	5
Inguinal hernia	6
Cryptorchidism	6
Urology	
Cohen's procedure in vesicoureteral reflux	12
Bladder reconstruction in bladder exstrophy	3
Excision of bladder diverticulum	1
Excision of bladder (after bladder exstrophy)	1
Cutaneous ureterostomy	3
Nephrectomy	1
Heminephrectomy	3
Bone surgery	
Juvenile bone cyst near humerus	2
Autologous spongiosaplasty (pelvis)	4
Osteotomy of pelvis (bladder exstrophy)	3
Biopsy of bone tumour (Ewing's sarcoma, osteosarcoma)	3
Neurosurgery	
Myelomeningocele	5
Hydrocephalus, Spitz-Holter shunt	3
Epidural haematoma	2
Insertion of Richmond screw	2
Tumour surgery	
Wilms' tumour	2
Resection of soft tissue tumour	2
Tumour biopsy	4

pel the blade and its thermal energy have to be used in such a manner that bleeding does not begin. This is done by making incisions at a somewhat slower cutting speed than with the cold scalpel or the Bovie scalpel. The incisions have to be done at a constant speed through thinner layers of tissue to maintain constant and meticulous haemostasis at every step. The cutting technique required for effective use of the Shaw scalpel was initially unfamiliar and the use of the instrument was therefore fully effective only after a short learning period. However, this change in technique was not difficult to achieve and much easier than that required for lasers. The time loss because of the lower cutting speed was more than compensated by the gain in time due to a dry operating field. For skin incisions, we usually used a temperature of 110°C. After cutting through the dermis, the blade

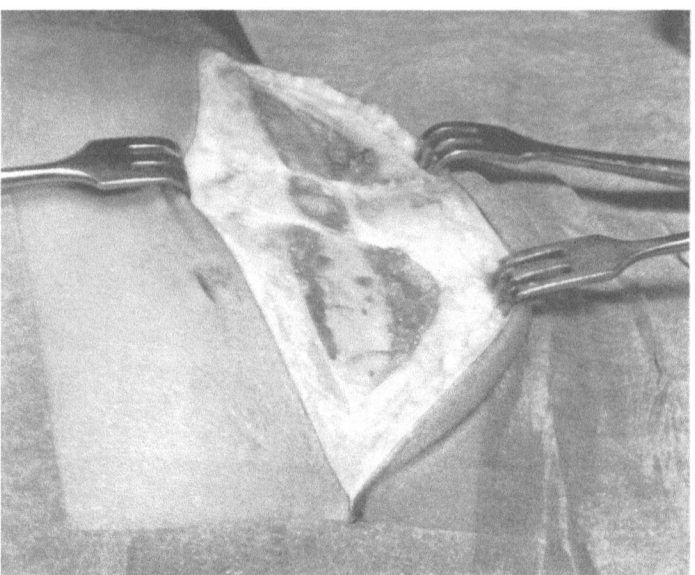

Fig. 3. Abdominal incision with the Shaw haemostatic scalpel; bloodless surgery

temperature was usually raised to 220°–260°C. The grade of haemostasis with these temperatures was usually excellent in subcutaneous and fibrous tissues and muscles. Of course, one has to adapt the speed carefully to the type and vascularity of the tissues at these high temperatures. However, with increasing experience this was not very difficult. The haemostasis achieved was usually excellent, especially in abdominal and thoracic wall incisions and after a short learning period, no additional electrosurgical unit (ESU) was used and only a few or no ligatures at all were necessary. Figure 3 shows a bloodless field in a patient with an upper abdominal transverse incision. The dry operating field gave much better visibility and was of considerable advantage to the surgeon.

Cutting through muscles could be done with more surgical precision because muscle stimulation associated with passing electric current through the body is eliminated. Since no electric current passes through the patient no grounding pad is necessary and the risk of accidental electrical burns at grounding sites is eliminated. This was of special interest for us in neonates and infants. Deep in the abdominal cavity, there was sometimes a slight mechanical inconvenience because of the cable on the proximal end of the scalpel handle. It is important to realize that if the ESU is used in conjunction with the Shaw scalpel, care must be taken not to touch the blade with the activated ESU as this would result in internal damage to the electronics in the Shaw controller unit. In minor procedures, usually one No. 10 or No. 15 blade was used, in major procedures two to four blades were necessary. The blades were mostly as sharp as normal cold steel blades and maintained their sharpness for about 20 min. However, there were a few blades which seemed to get dull more quickly and a few which seemed not to be as sharp as normal cold blades initially. A few trials to resterilize the blades were unsuccessful because they got dull. We initially thought that the Shaw haemostatic scalpel would also be advantageous in surgery on the liver and spleen. However, we were not very successful with this system on these parenchymatous organs because of too much coagulated blood on the blades, in spite of the Teflon coating.

Altogether, the Shaw haemostatic scalpel proved to be useful in about four-fifths of our operations. The immediate haemostasis, allowing for increased visibility in the operative field, and the lack of muscle stimulation, allowing more precise cutting, was a considerable advantage in all major operations and was of course of special interest in neonatal surgery. In this field, perfect haemostasis and excellent visibility of the operative field is especially important. We also had the impression that, in comparison with conventional ESU, there was less tissue damage with the haemostatic scalpel. In contradiction to reports on adults, we have the impression that the quantity of fluid administered was not greatly influenced by the use of the Shaw scalpel, mainly because meticulous operative haemostasis is mandatory in paediatric surgery anyway. However, haemostasis was much more easy to achieve and in some extensive procedures we also think that the quantity of blood administered was reduced. In very major procedures, the operative time seemed to be reduced; in none of the procedures was it longer than with conventional techniques.

Wound Healing

There was one infection of an abdominal wall incision with partial disruption of the wound on day 14 in an infant with hepatoportoenterostomy (Kimura–Kasai procedure) because of biliary atresia. One patient had a slight seroma which healed without sequelae, in three patients the incision was red from day 2 to day 4 which could be explained by too low a speed of skin or subcutaneous tissue incision, resulting in slight thermal injury. However, wound healing was subsequently normal in these patients. All other patients had completely uneventful postoperative courses, normal wound healing and the cosmetic appearance of the scar at late follow-up was good and equivalent to incisions with the cold scalpel. The complication rate of wound healing was similar to the complication rate with the cold steel scalpel.

Discussion

Our first series of 100 operations with the Shaw haemostatic scalpel convinced us of the advantages of this new technique and the Shaw scalpel is now successfully used by all senior members of our staff. Controlled experimental animal studies were conducted during 1978 and 1979 by Stanley M. Levenson, Professor of Surgery, Albert Einstein College of Medicine, New York, a recognized authority on wound healing [3]. Levenson compared postoperative wound breaking strength in standard paramedian incisions in rats. The incisions were made with an ordinary scalpel, the heated Shaw haemostatic scalpel and the conventional ESU unit, with both coagulation and cutting. Wound healing and breaking strength were tested between 7 and 42 days postoperatively. They were proved to be highest in incisions made with the conventional scalpel and the thermally regulated Shaw haemostatic scalpel. At day 21 there was a slight difference in favour of the conventional scalpel which was, however, not demonstrable later on. Both the conventional scalpel and the Shaw scalpel produced less tissue damage than incisions made with the ESU and there was no instance of wound infection in any of the rats of the whole series. The conventional scalpel and the Shaw scalpel produced statistically stronger wounds than incisions made with the ESU in either its coagulation or cutting mode. Wound resistance to infection after incisions with the Shaw scalpel and the conventional scalpel by purposely inoculated skin incisions in rats up to 10^8 *Pseudomonas aeruginosa* or *Staphylococcus aureus* did not show any difference between the conventional scalpel and the Shaw scalpel at various temperatures. No wound infection developed in either group.

Levenson also compared the cold scalpel and the thermally regulated haemostatic scalpel for excision of third-degree burns in Hampshire–Landrace pigs [4]. He found that the blood loss was significantly less than in comparable excisions carried out with the usual "cold" surgical scalpel and the "takes" of immediately applied skin grafts were similar following excision with the cold surgical scalpel. He was then the first to apply the Shaw haemostatic scalpel successfully in a 50-year-old man with 35% third-degree burns [4]. Since then, favourable reports have been published by different authors from many fields of surgery [1, 2, 5–10]. Salyer [7] reported on its use in plastic and reconstructive surgery, especially in craniomaxillofacial surgery and cleft palate surgery. Pilnik and co-workers [6] reported on the use of the haemostatic scalpel in operations on the breast, pointing out especially the reduction of blood loss. None of their 155 mastectomies done with the heated scalpel required a single blood transfusion. Fee [2] reported on 25 patients who underwent parotid gland surgery with the Shaw scalpel and compared this group of patients with another group of 25 patients who had similar surgery by conventional techniques. Overall, the patients operated on with the Shaw scalpel had less blood loss and shorter operative times. In addition, in patients who underwent superficial parotidectomy, the incidence of temporary partial facial nerve paralysis was lower with the Shaw scalpel. They concluded that the Shaw haemostatic scalpel was a safe efficacious instrument for use in parotid gland surgery. These authors especially stress the better visibility due to the dry operative field. Fee [1] also reported on the use of the Shaw scalpel in head and neck surgery and classified the procedures in 50 patients on a scoring system for effectiveness of haemostasis. Subjective equipment evaluation resulted in a mean score of 3.8 (1 = worthless, 5 = excellent). Overall, the Shaw system was a worthwhile surgical tool in over 70% of cases. The author stresses that the Shaw scalpel system is especially excellent for raising flaps and for use in precise surgery where small capillary bleeding typically obscures visibility, especially in parotid surgery.

Moazed and co-workers [5] reported on the use of the Shaw haemostatic scalpel in ophthalmic surgery. They also stress the preservation of a good view of the anatomy during dissection and come to the conclusion that the Shaw scalpel simplifies operative procedures at the orbit and the lid. They also noted a significant shortening of surgical procedures in their ten cases. Tromovitch and co-workers [10] used the Shaw haemostatic scalpel in 150 minor and major dermatological procedures. They state that "the dissection and control of bleeding was infinitely easier" with the Shaw scalpel and that "this electric scalpel will surely become a favourite instrument for dermatological surgeons". Takagi and co-workers [9] used the Shaw haemostatic scalpel in 7 radical operations for oral cancer and compared the amount of bleeding and postoperative exudate and the occurrence of postoperative complications with that from 12 operations performed with the conventional steel scalpel. The blood loss during the radical neck dissection procedure performed with the Shaw scalpel was 39% of the control value, and no blood transfusions were necessary.

We add our own experience with over 3000 cases with the Shaw haemostatic scalpel to these favourable reports in the literature. We would like to stress again the advantages which are especially important in paediatric surgery. The Shaw scalpel allows one to seal small vessels with heat as it cuts, largely eliminating the flow of blood into the incised area and giving an improved visibility and a dry operative field. Since no electric current travels through the patient, there is no disturbing excitation of muscles, allowing for more precise cutting. There is also no earthing pad required which eliminates the potential danger of electrical burns. Improved visibility, reduced tissue damage, lack of muscle stimulation and the elimination of possible electrical burns are of special interest for the paediatric surgeon. After a short training in cutting techniques, the use of the Shaw haemostatic scalpel, facilitate greatly haemostasis, another important factor in young patients.

References

1. Fee WE (1981) Use of the Shaw scalpel in head and neck surgery. Otolaryngol Head Neck Surg 89:515–519
2. Fee WE (1984) Parotid gland surgery – using the Shaw hemostatic scalpel. Arch Otolaryngol 110:739–741
3. Levenson SM, Kan-Gruber D, Gruber C, et al (1979) Effect of a new heated scalpel (Shaw) on the healing of skin incisions of rats. Paper presented at the annual meeting of the Halsted Society, Little Rock, AR, Oct 5
4. Levenson SM, Kan-Gruber D, Gruber C, Seifter E, Molnar J, Petro J (1982) A hemostatic scalpel for burn debridement. Arch Surg 117:213–220
5. Moazed KT, Trokel SL (1983) Use of the Shaw scalpel in ophthalmic surgery. Ophthalmic Surg 14:432–434
6. Pilnik S, Steichen F (1986) The use of the hemostatic scalpel in operations upon the breast. Surg Gynecol Obstet 162:589–591
7. Salyer KE (1984) Use of a new hemostatic scalpel in plastic surgery. Ann Plast Surg 13:532–538
8. Steichen FM, Levenson SM (1985) The Shaw hemostatic scalpel. Probl Gen Surg 2:11–17
9. Takagi R, Ohashi Y, Abe M (1985) Blood loss with use of the Shaw scalpel for the treatment of oral cancer. J Oral Maxillofac Surg 43:580–584
10. Tromovitch TA, Glogau RG, Stegman SJ (1983) The Shaw scalpel. J Dermatol Surg Oncol 9:316–319

Liver Resection with the Sonocut Ultrasonic Knife

B. Thomasson[1], L. Hedenborg[2], and H. Wiksell[3]

Summary

Previous reports and our findings suggest that resection by ultrasound is of appreciable merit in liver surgery. Blood can be saved and bile leakage diminished as the larger vessels and bile ducts can be skeletonized unharmed, whereas the dissector selectively carries away the parenchyma. Otherwise virtually inaccessible tumours can be approached. The ultrasonic dissector/aspirator does not harm the tissue in depth beyond the resection surface and thus not much devitalized tissue is left in the wound.

Zusammenfassung

Berichte aus der Literatur und eigene Erfahrungen zeigen, daß die Ultraschallresektion von beträchtlichem Wert in der Leberchirurgie ist. Es kann blutsparend operiert werden, Gallelecks werden verringert, da größere Gefäße und Gallengänge sorgfältig präpariert werden, während der Ultraschalldissektor selektiv das Leberparenchym abträgt. Sonst inoperable Tumoren können somit chirurgisch angegangen werden. Der Ultraschalldissektor/-aspirator läßt das tiefe Gewebe jenseits der Resektionsebene unangetastet, wodurch nur sehr wenig devitalisiertes Gewebe zurückbleibt.

Résumé

Nous voulons montrer, à travers notre expérience et à la lumière de la littérature médicale, l'intérêt majeur du bistouri à ultrason en chirurgie hépatologique. Il permet une intervention peu sanglante, minimise une fuite biliaire car les gros vaisseaux sanguins, de même que les canaux hépatiques sont particulièrement bien préparés pendant l'utilisation du bistouri à ultrason sur le parenchyme hépatique. Des tumeurs non accessibles à la chirurgie en temps ordinaire le deviennent. Grâce à cet instrument, il n'y aura aucune atteinte du tissu sous-jacent et donc très peu d'atteintes nerveuses.

Introduction

A potentially dangerous feature associated with resection of parenchymatous organs is the frequently excessive blood loss. Although exsanguination can usually be avoided, the loss generally necessitates large transfusions with their inherent

[1] Department of Paediatric Surgery, Karolinska Institute, Stockholm, Sweden
[2] Department of Pathology, St. Göran's Hospital, Stockholm, Sweden
[3] Royal Institute of Technology and Ingenjörsfirma Comair AB, Stockholm, Sweden

dangers. In liver resections leakage of bile further enhances the risk of complications.

Accordingly, continuous efforts have been made to develop new techniques aiming to facilitate the procedures, to save blood and to prevent bile leakage [1, 4–6, 9–15]. One of the newer modalities in this respect is utilization of ultrasonic energy for resection. The concept of phacoemulsification was introduced in ophthalmic surgery in the late 1960s [8]. The technique was then modified for use in other tissues (brain, liver, pancreas) and employed in clinical neurosurgery about 10 years later [3].

To date at least four devices have been made available: Camtom (Heidelberg, Federal Republic of Germany), Cavitron (Mountain View, California, United States), Sonocut (Stockholm, Sweden) and Sonotec (Tokyo, Japan) (Hodgson et al. 1987, unpublished data; [2]). The Sonocut was designed by one of us (H.W.) in 1985. So far 79 units have been produced and they have been used in about 2000 operations in various countries. The first clinical application of this device was for resection of brain tumours at the beginning of 1986 at the Department of Neurosurgery, Karolinska Hospital, Stockholm [16].

Technical Description

The main console of the unit comes in two versions, the Maxi (Fig. 1) and the Mini (Fig. 2). The Maxi type is completely self-contained, including suction and irrigation, whereas the appreciably less expensive Mini has to be attached to an exter-

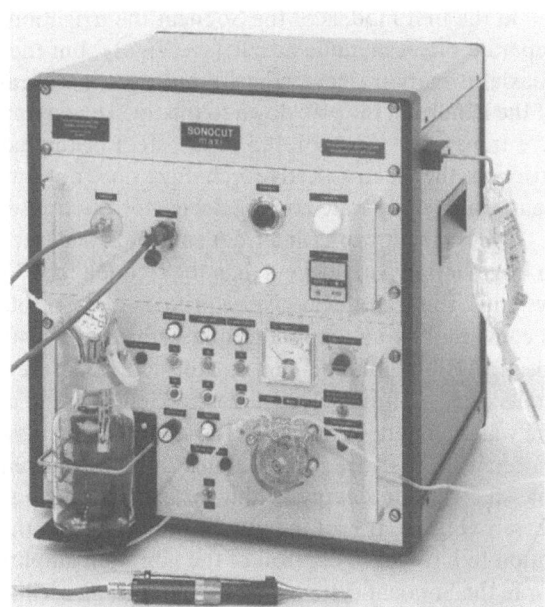

Fig. 1. The Sonocut Maxi console, incorporating irrigation and suction devices. Straight handle with offset metallic irrigation nozzle

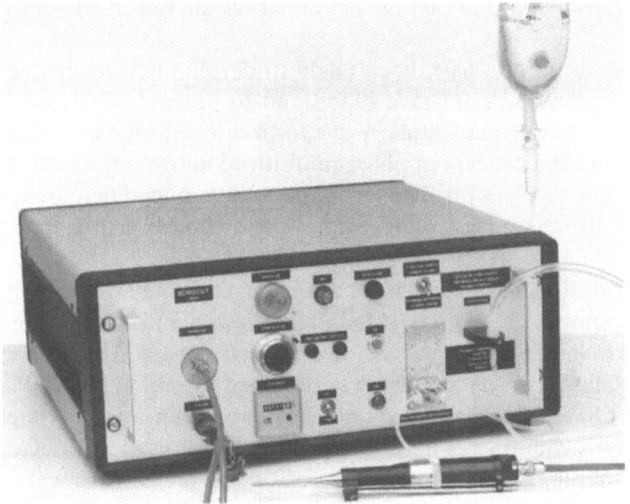

Fig. 2. The Sonocut Mini console. This version contains the electrostrictive power plant only. External irrigation and suction are needed

nal suction device and uses irrigation by gravity. Both types of console activate identical handles. These are available in straight or bent versions and can be autoclaved at 135°C. They are insulated in accordance with IEC 601-1 cardiac floating standard to allow the use of monopolar electrocautery. The angulated handpiece facilitates operation in the narrow field of an operating microscope.

In the first models of the Sonocut the irrigation fluid was dispersed through a separate offset metallic nozzle (see Fig. 1), but the provision of a nonconducting coaxial irrigation sleeve (Fig. 3) improves the ultrasonic and electrical insulation of the handle all the way down to the tip. The energy is provided by an electrostrictive transducer incorporated in the stem of the handle. In contrast to magnetostriction, the electrostrictive technique does not waste much energy in the form of heat. Thus, a separate cooling device for the transducer is not necessary.

The Sonocut works at a frequency of 24000 Hz, which is slightly more efficient in fragmenting parenchyma than the frequency of 35000 Hz utilized by some other systems. The transducer gives a primary acoustic output of 15 µm maximally. This is converted by an amplitude transformer to 5–240 µm longitudinal vibrations of the tip. The amplitude can be adjusted while the device is running. Within the limits of 30–150 µm selective destruction of tissue can be achieved, depending on the water content of the cells. Those containing more water (e.g. hepatocytes) are more easily destroyed than tissues such as collagen and elastin (e.g. vessels and bile ducts). The energy at the tip is dispersed purely longitudinally, not transversely (Fig. 4). It is of the utmost importance to the selectivity of tissue fragmentation to have strict controll of the vibration amplitude of the tip. A phase detector in the Sonocut system enables the feeding oscillator to maintain a stable acoustic output irrespective of changing workloads.

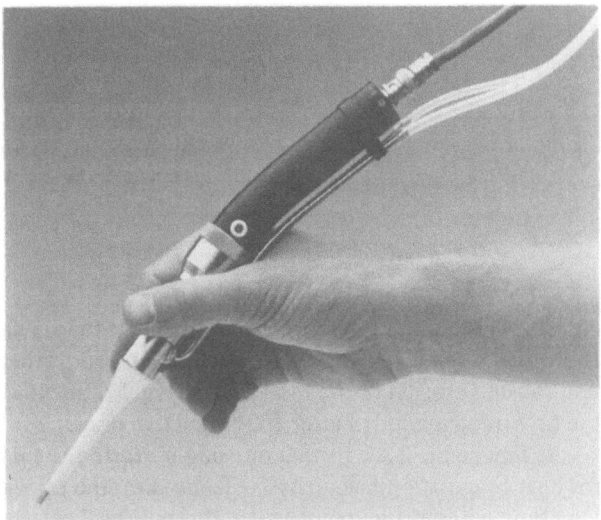

Fig. 3. Angulated handle with coaxial irrigation sleeve

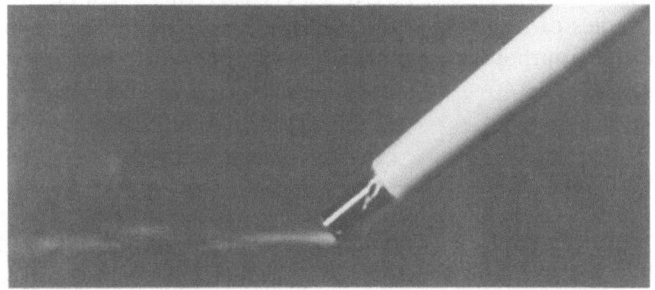

Fig. 4. The tip in action, demonstrating the strictly longitudinal energy distribution. The drop of irrigation fluid coming out of the coaxial irrigation sleeve is undisturbed as long as it is hanging at the side of the metal tip, whereas it is nebulized when it reaches the front of the tip

The titanium alloy tip is provided with a central 2 mm diameter suction channel. Irrigation is provided by sterile isotonic saline 5–35 ml/min. The suction can be adjusted from 0 to −0.8 bar. The fragmentation of tissue is so efficient that obstruction of the suction channel hardly ever occurs. Utilization of fruit or vegetables as test or training material for the Sonocut is, however, unwise. Many fruit contain seeds, which may obstruct the suction channel. Cutting into plastic material is still worse. The plastic melts at the tip and resets into hard plugs in the channel. A piece of liver is recommended as training material.

High frequency vibrations are known to cause fatigue fractures in metal. In the Sonocut tip the maximum mechanical strain occurs 2–3 cm from the point. However, even during prolonged (200 h) endurance tests no stress fractures have oc-

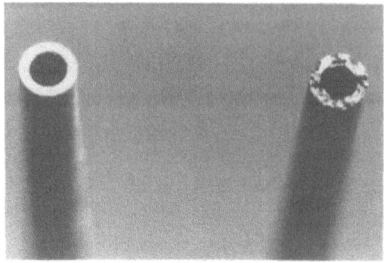

Fig. 5. On the left an unused Sonocut metal tip, on the right another tip after 200 h of active operation at maximal vibration amplitude against a water surface. The cavitation is clearly noticeable. The diameter of the central suction channel is 2 mm

curred. At the vibration frequencies and amplitudes employed, the limiting factor is not the Wöhler stress fracture correlation, but rather the cavitation phenomenon causing erosion of the metallic tip (Fig. 5). In clinical practice replacement of the tip is recommended after 100 h of active usage.

At first sight, it seems that one might utilize the tip of the ultrasonic aspirator for heat coagulation haemostasis. To be sure, the tip will heat up if operated for a long time without suction or irrigation, but this heat energy cannot be easily controlled for haemostasis [7]. Furthermore, the temperature might damage the rather expensive tip. As mentioned earlier the Sonocut handle is nevertheless designed for monopolar electrocautery use. This might not necessarily apply to the handles of some other ultrasonic knives. Before utilization of such for electrocautery purposes the manufacturer of the actual ultrasonic device should be consulted.

Clinical Experience

We have tested the Sonocut Maxi in the experimental laboratory and employed it in five cases of liver resection for primary and metastatic liver tumours in children (ages 2–16 years) at the Department of Paediatric Surgery, St. Göran's Hospital. This, of course, is a very limited experience, but the versatility of ultrasonic dissection has been impressive and was thought to warrant a report. In the patients with metastases multiple lesions were removed. The majority of the cases were further complicated because the tumours involved other organs as well (adrenal gland, lung, stomach) so that the operations were reoperations in scarred fields. The procedures ranged from local tumour enucleations to right lobectomy. The children all survived the operations, but two have recurrent metastatic disease (one girl in the liver and another disseminated in multiple organs).

It was found that the difference in texture between tumour tissue and normal liver was great enough to allow for an easy, clean dissection along the tumour capsule without breaking it. Likewise, larger vessels and bile ducts were skeletonized, but remained intact and could easily be individually obliterated by cautery, silver clips or ligature (Figs. 6 and 7). In one case a large tumour was located close to the liver hilus in the medial left lobe of the liver. We feel that we would not have been able to accomplish complete removal of the tumour, with the capsule intact

6 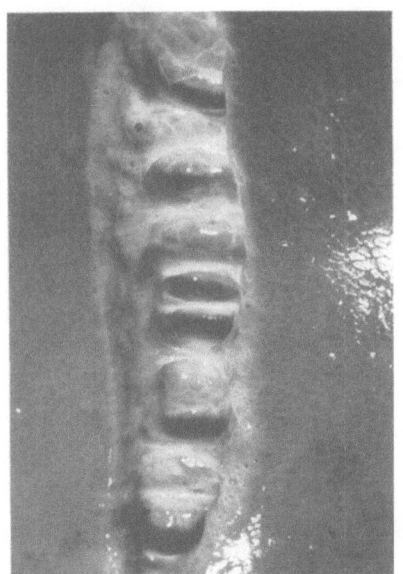 7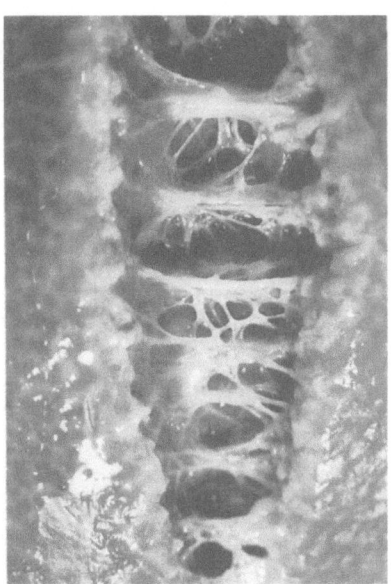

Fig. 6. Liver resection in vitro. Note the intact skeletonized vessels and bile ducts bridging the gap created in the parenchyma by ultrasonic dissection/aspiration

Fig. 7. Spleen resection in vitro. Note the "cleaned" bridging vessels

and without breaking into the closely adjacent large vessels and bile ducts without the aid of the ultrasonic dissector.

However, in another case with some fibrosis of the liver the properties of the tumour and the surrounding liver tissue differed very little. A very fine adjustment of the vibration amplitude of the dissector tip was necessary in this case in order to achieve selective tissue destruction. In some areas the energy necessary to remove parenchyma was high enough to cause unpleasantly profuse bleeding.

The ultrasonic procedure is facilitated by manual fixation of the tissue to be dissected, e.g. by applying a stretching force to the liver lobe in question. The liver capsule in all cases demonstrated tough resistance to the ultrasonic aspirator. It was found most convenient to start the dissection by incising the capsule with an ordinary scalpel. Even with the Sonocut the blood loss was considerable in all five operations, on average 60% (range 20%–120%) of the patient's blood volume. It is our impression, however, that compared with earlier operations of similar magnitude the ultrasonic dissector saved considerable amounts of blood.

Histological Studies

Liver tissue resected by ultrasound or an ordinary electrocautery knife from pigs and by ultrasound from a patient was studied by light microscopy. The tissue was

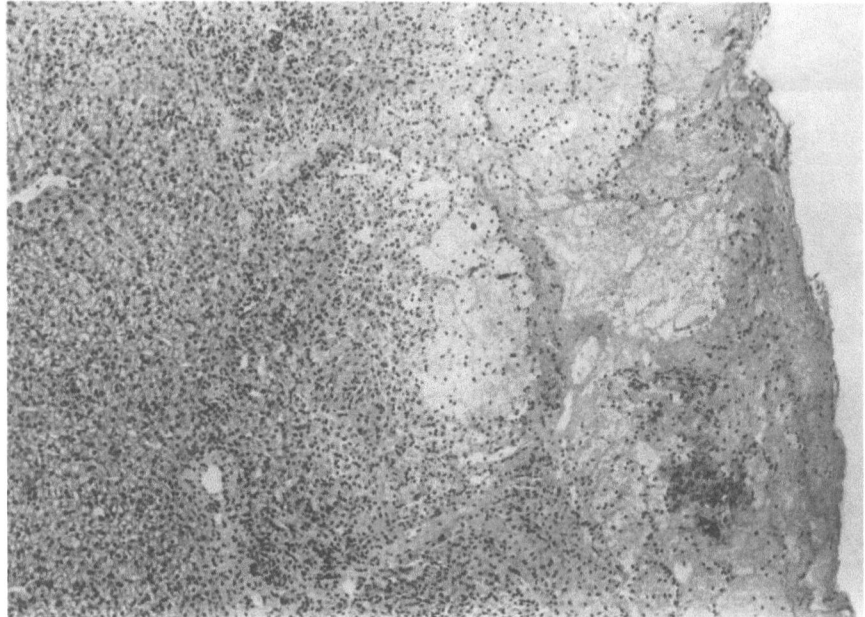

Fig. 8. Ultrasonically resected hepatic tissue from a pig. The illustration shows a zone of approximately 1.5 mm with the resection surface to the right. The surface is covered by coagulated material. Tissue on the right-hand side of the picture shows degenerated and destroyed hepatocytes. In the middle there are slight cystic changes with granulocytes, erythrocytes and fibrin. Histologically normal hepatocytes appear to the left at a depth of approximately 1 mm. H & E, × 90

fixed in 10% formalin, processed according to standard routine, embedded in paraffin and stained by haematoxylin-eosin and van Gieson stain.

Resection of liver from pigs (Fig. 8) by ultrasound resulted in similar morphological findings compared with the damage caused by the ordinary cautery knife. Histological changes were seen in a narrow zone from the resection surface, 0.5–2 mm deep. Hepatocytes showed polygonal eosinophilic cytoplasm with a granular appearance. Separation of liver cell trabeculae and widening of sinusoidal spaces, together with accumulation of erythrocytes, was noted. Nuclear changes consisted of slight pyknosis and hyperchromasia together with a tendency to elongation suggestive of electro-artefacts.

In some areas irregular cystic spaces had developed, empty or filled with fluid, coated by a thin layer of coagulated cellular material. The size of the cysts varied from approximately 100 to 500 μm. Aggregations of granulocytes under the partly coagulated resection surface and at the border with normal liver tissue were seen. In the vicinity of connective tissue septa and vessels one could see cellular changes, small haemorrhages and exudation of fibrin to a depth of 2 mm. The plane of resection often seemed to follow the normal lobular architecture of the liver.

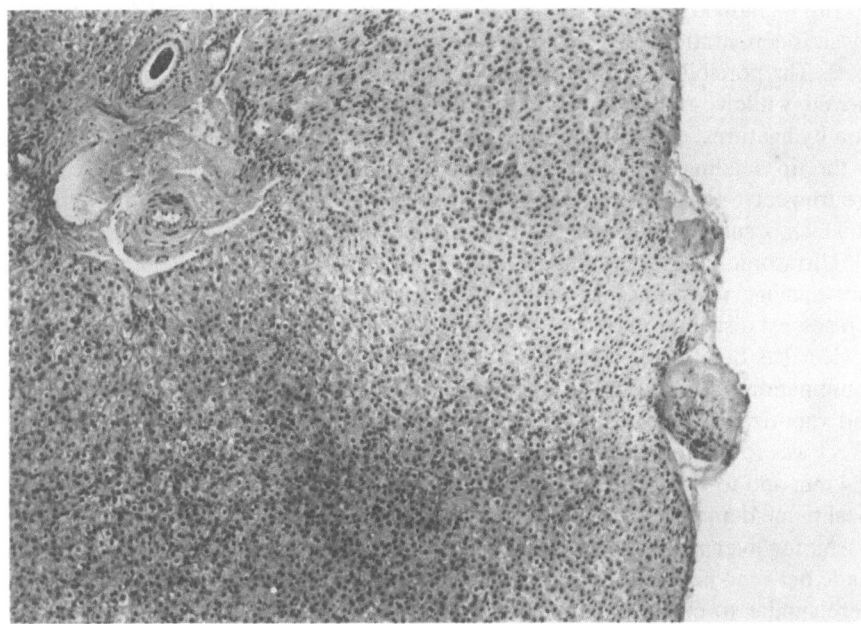

Fig. 9. Ultrasonically resected hepatic tissue from a patient. The illustration shows a zone of approximately 1.5 mm with the resection surface to the right. In the upper left-hand corner there is a small portal zone, on the surface a thin layer of coagulated material. The hepatic tissue in the upper right-hand corner has a more eosinophilic cytoplasm (paler in the picture) and nuclear changes (pyknosis, hyperchromasia). In the portal zone and just under the surface there is accumulation of erythrocytes. The depth of histological changes is approximately 1 mm. H & E, × 90

Our impression is that there was no significant difference in histological findings in pig liver resected by ultrasound compared with resection by the cautery knife. The resection surface from the patient (Fig. 9) showed the same kind of changes as the material from pigs, even if the tissue damage in the patient's tissues was less pronounced. This might be due to the fact that the ultrasonic dissector was tuned somewhat more "boldly" in the experimental than in the clinical setting.

Discussion

The ultrasonic aspirator has two unique properties making it especially attractive in liver surgery:

1. The ability to resect tissue with accuracy, deep within a cramped operation area with only very small movements of the handle and with tip vibrations restricted to micrometres. This is possibly due to the enormous acceleration of the

tip (up to 340 000 g) causing an acoustic "impedance catastrophe" and resulting in tissue fragmentation.

2. The possibility of selective tissue destruction. Thus, parenchyma can be removed, while vessels and bile ducts remain intact and available for selective occlusion by ligatures, clips or cautery. This is dependent on a cavitation phenomenon at the tip, leading to so-called rectified diffusion. Gases dissolved in body fluids are transferred into the gaseous phase causing cellular ruptures, a larger number of which occur the higher the water content of the tissue.

Ultrasonic aspirators should not be utilized in the bones of the cranium. Distant damage to cranial nerves has been reported, probably caused by massive transosseal distribution of the ultrasound energy. The cutting effect of ultrasound devices has been studied histologically in laboratory animals and described as a combination of cavitation (rupture of cell structures), an adiabatic heating effect and vaporization of cell liquid. In a report by Boddy et al. [2] the local heating effect was found to be limited to a rise in temperature by $17°-18°C$ at a distance of 1 mm and to $3°-4°C$ at a distance of 3 mm from the tip of the scalpel. Minimal local tissue damage and healing without fibrosis was recorded.

As for liver resection there is a study in dogs where a comparison has been made between laser, ultrasound and blunt dissection [15]. Laser-induced changes were similar to our lesions induced by ultrasound and located at a depth of approximately 3 mm. In the report changes induced by ultrasound were limited to 1 mm and by blunt dissection to 0.5 mm. In spite of this the blunt dissection animals showed more extensive postoperative necrosis after 7 days. Laser resection was followed by a higher degree of local infection. The authors stress the combination of gentler handling of the tissue and clearer visualization of anatomical structures with the use of ultrasound for resection. Also in the animal experiments performed by Ottow et al. [11], the ultrasonic technique combined a tendency towards smaller blood loss with minimal tissue necrosis. Our findings are in good accordance with these two reports as we find only minimal tissue changes in a narrow zone of 0.5–2 mm. The variability in the findings can be explained by the fact that different amounts of energy were used during the operations.

References

1. Andrus CH, Kaminski DL (1986) Segmental hepatic resection utilizing the ultrasonic dissector. Arch Surg 121:515–521
2. Boddy S-AM, Ramsay JWA, Carter SSC, Webster PJR, Levison DA, Whitfield HN (1987) Tissue effects of an ultrasonic scalpel for clinical surgical use. Urol Res 15:49–52
3. Flamm ES, Ransohoff J, Wuchinich D, Broadwin A (1978) Preliminary experience with ultrasonic aspiration in neurosurgery. Neurosurgery 2:240–245
4. Goldsmith NA, Woodburne RT (1957) The surgical anatomy pertaining to liver resection. Surg Gynecol Obstet 105:310–318
5. Hodgson WJB (1979) The ultrasonic scalpel. Bull NY Acad Med 55:908–915
6. Hodgson WJB, DelGuercio LRM (1984) Preliminary experience in liver surgery using the ultrasonic scalpel. Surgery 95:230–234

7. Hodgson WJB, Poddar PK, Mencer EJ, Wiliams J, Drew M, McElhinney AJ (1979) Evaluation of ultrasonically powered instruments in the laboratory and in the clinical setting. Am J Gastroenterol 72:133–140

8. Kelman CD (1969) Phaco-emulsification and aspiration. Am J Ophthalmol 67:464–477

9. Lin T-Y (1973) Results in 107 hepatic lobectomies with a preliminary report on the use of a clamp to reduce blood loss. Ann Surg 177:413–421

10. Makuuchi M, Hasegawa H, Yamazaki S, Takayasu K (1987) Four new hepatectomy procedures for resection of the right hepatic vein and preservation of the inferior right hepatic vein. Surg Gynecol Obstet 164:69–72

11. Ottow RT, Barbieri SA, Sugarbaker PH, Wesley RA (1985) Liver transection: a controlled study of four different techniques in pigs. Surgery 97:596–601

12. Pachter HL, Spencer FC, Hofstetter SR, Coppa GF (1983) Experience with the finger fracture technique to achieve intra-hepatic hemostasis in 75 patients with severe injuries of the liver. Ann Surg 197:771–778

13. Putnam CW (1983) Techniques of ultrasonic dissection in resection of the liver. Surg Gynecol Obstet 157:474–478

14. Starzl TE, Bell RH, Beart RW, Putnam CW (1975) Hepatic trisegmentectomy and other liver resections. Surg Gynecol Obstet 141:429–437

15. Tranberg K-G, Rigotti P, Brackett KA, Bjornson HS, Fischer JE, Joffe SN (1986) Liver resection. A comparison using the Nd-YAG laser, an ultrasonic surgical aspirator, or blunt dissection. Am J Surg 151:368–373

16. Wiksell H, Granholm L (1986) Utveckling av ett nytt system för användning vid bl a tumöroperationer (Development of a new system for surgical ultrasonic aspiration). Lakartidningen 83:3990–3993

Electroresection
with a New Endotracheally Applicable Resectoscope

W. Geissler, K. Körner, and P. Wurnig

Summary

Besides dilatation, cryotherapy, laser and surgical resection, the technique of endoscopic, endotracheal electroresection provides an alternative in the treatment of endotracheal stenoses. The instrument is similar to the resectoscope used in urology, but additionally equipped with a longer action range and respiration facility. It is insulated at the tip of the shaft.

The electroresectoscope was employed on 64 occasions at our institution in three indications: endotracheal diseases, granulomas following tracheostomy; and short subglottic membrane stenoses, partly secondary to long-term intubation. Indications, advantages and drawbacks of the method are discussed.

Zusammenfassung

Neben Bougierung, Kryotherapie, Laser and operativer Resektion stellt die endoskopische, endotracheale Elektroresektion ein alternatives Verfahren zur Behandlung endotrachealer Stenosen dar. Das Gerät ähnelt dem in der Urologie verwendeten Resektoskop, weist jedoch eine größere Arbeitslänge und eine Beatmungsmöglichkeit auf. Es ist an der Spitze des Schafts isoliert.

Seit 1985 wurde es 64mal bei 3 Erkrankungsgruppen verwendet, und zwar bei 1) endotrachealen Veränderungen, 2) Granulombildung bei Kanülenträgern und 3) kurzstreckigen subglottischen Membranstenosen, z. T. nach Langzeitintubation. Die Indikationen sowie Vor- und Nachteile des Verfahrens werden diskutiert.

Résumé

A côté des dilatations par bougies, de la cryothérapie, du laser et des résections chirurgicales, l'électrosection endotrachéale par endoscopic représente une alternative intéressante dans les traitement de la sténose trachéale. Cet instrument est très voisin d'un résecteur urologique mais dispose en plus d'un prolongateur et d'un respirateur. L'extrémité de l'appareil est isolée. Depuis 1985, nous l'avons utilisé dans 64 cas, dans 3 types de séries. 1ère série: pathologie endotrachéale, 2ème série: lors de granulomes sur canules de trachéotomie, 3ème série: lors de sténoses sous-glottiques membraneuses après intubation de longue durée. Nous discuterons les indications pré- et post-opératoires.

Introduction

Therapeutic problems may arise in endotracheal stenoses in infancy because of the small dimensions. Resection with end-to-end anastomosis, laser resection,

Mautner Markhofsches Kinderspital der Stadt Wien, Baumgasse 75, 1030 Vienna, Austria

Progress in Pediatric Surgery, Vol. 25
Angerpointner (Ed.)
© Springer-Verlag Berlin Heidelberg 1990

electroresection, dilatation or tracheal enlargement by chondroplasty modified according to Hof [10] are all possibilities for treatment. We have already reported on these methods [8, 15, 18, 19]. In this paper a resection device is presented which is particularly suited to the small tracheal stenoses in infancy.

Method

Since 1985 the resection device shown in Fig. 1 has been available for electroresection (produced by Storz, D-7200 Tuttlingen, Federal Republic of Germany). Simultaneous ventilation during resection is possible. It is small enough to be used

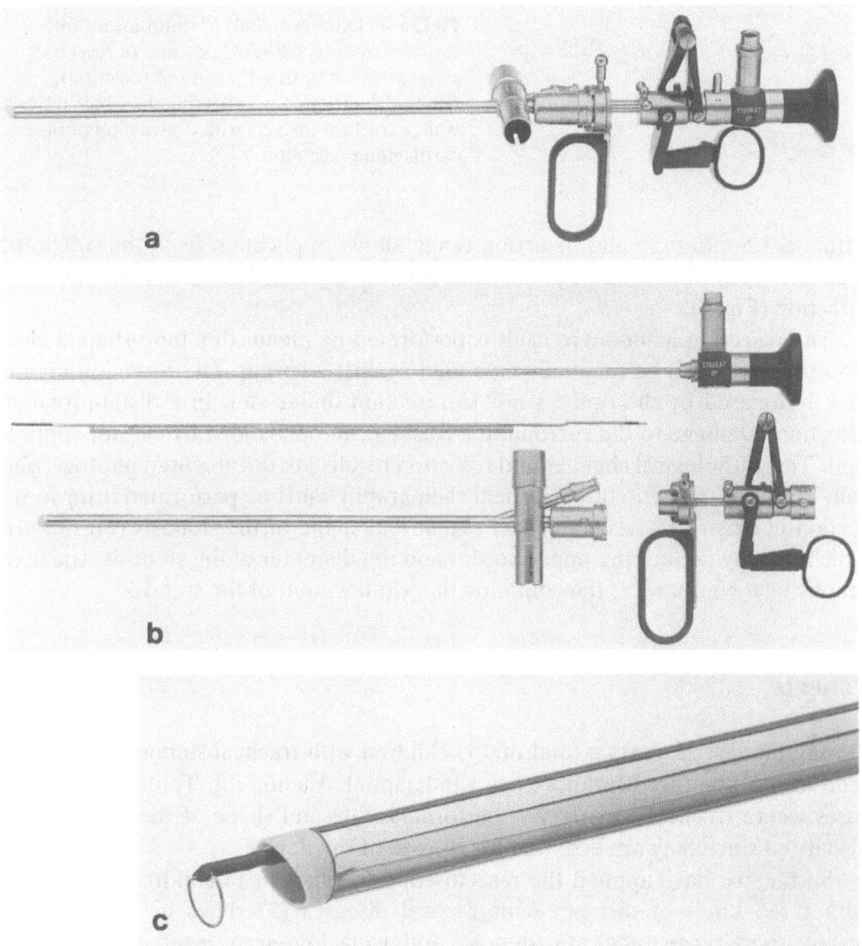

Fig. 1a–c. Resection device for endotracheal and endobronchial resection with ventilation socket. **a** overall view, **b** individual parts (top: optics; middle: resection electrode; bottom: shaft with ventilation socket; right : resection handle), **c** insulated shaft top with extended resection sling

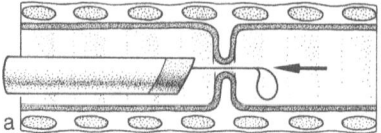

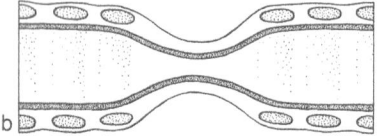

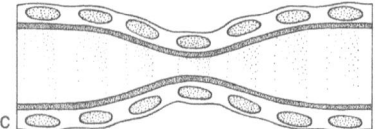

Fig. 2a–c. Different kinds of stenoses. **a** short-distance stenosis (showing position of resection sling; *arrow* indicates direction of resection), **b** long-distance stenosis affecting the whole tracheal wall, **c** tracheal malacia with destruction of the cartilaginous skeleton

within a 3.5-mm tube and its action range allows application from the subglottic region down to the carina. Resection under view is carried out in a distal-proximal direction (Fig. 2).

The resection manoeuvre itself is performed by means of a loop-shaped electrotome which can be manually extended against a spring. The resection area is exactly focused by the optics prior to resection under view in a distal-proximal direction. Damage to the surrounding trachea can be avoided by careful application. The pathological changes and resection results are documented photographically. Besides tracheoscopy, tracheal radiography must be performed prior to resection in order to assess the exact extent and shape of the stenosis (Fig. 3a–d). Tracheoscopy defines the upper border and the diameter of the stenosis, tracheography its lower border, thus defining the whole extent of the stenosis.

Patients

During the last 25 years a total of 153 children with tracheal stenoses have been seen at the Mautner Markhofsches Kinderspital, Vienna [8]. Table 1 lists those cases where tracheal surgery was performed. Site and shape of the stenoses are also listed since they are essential for the use of the device.

So far, we have applied the resectoscope 64 times in 14 children, essentially with three kinds of disease: endotracheal diseases (37 times in 14 children); scarry, short-range subglottic stenoses following long-term intubation (method employed as supplementary or transitory measure prior to enlargement chondroplasty); and development of granulation tissue secondary to tracheostomy (14 times in 7 children). Three cases are presented in detail.

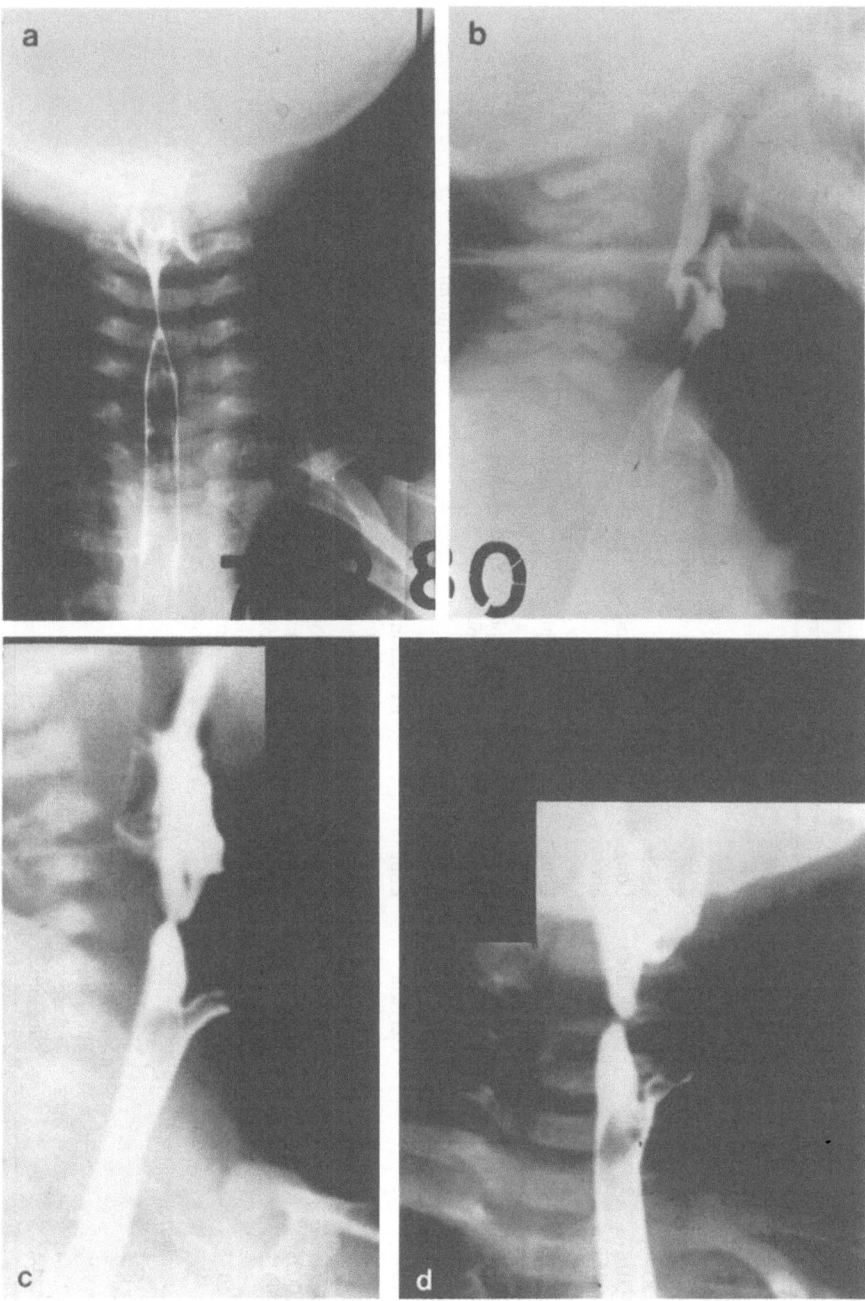

Fig. 3a–d. Tracheography for assessment of stenotic extent. **a, b** long-distance stenosis (case 12), **c, d** short-distance stenosis (case 3). Only this kind of stenosis is suited for electroresection

Table 1. Review of tracheal stenoses and procedures employed

Aetiology	Site	Type/histology	Operation	Laser	Electroresection	Dilatation
I. Iatrogenic						
a) Following long-term intubation						
1. 21094	Subglottic	Short			1 ×[a]	60 ×
2. 25061	Subglottic	Short				15 ×
3. 13000	Subglottic	Short			3 × (2 ×[a])	43 ×
4. 10018	Subglottic	Long	Tracheoplasty		1 ×[a]	
5. 19525	Subglottic	Short		2 ×		52 ×
6. 23639	Subglottic	Short			3 ×	
7. 22331	Subglottic	Long	Tracheoplasty	Repeated		
8. 1401/86	Subglottic	Long			23 ×	
9. 29422	Subglottic	Short	Tracheoplasty			10 ×
10. 87	Subglottic	Long	Tracheoplasty		Repeated resection of granulomas	
b) Following tracheostomy						
11. 21098	Cervical	Long	Resection + anastomosis			
II. Congenital						
12. 2291	Subglottic	Long	2 × Tracheoplasty		7 ×[a]	28 ×
13. 10005	Subglottic	Short	Tracheoplasty			
14. 19523	Subglottic	Long	Tracheoplasty		Repeated resection of granulomas	
15. 21097	Thoracic	Short	Resection + anastomosis			
III. Endotracheal disease						
16. 21583	Subglottic	Viral papilloma			3 ×	
17. 25986	Subglottic	Membranous			2 ×	
18. 21586	Subglottic	Polypal			1 ×	
19. 27314	Diffuse	Viral papilloma		Repeated	31 ×	
20. 28844	Subglottic	Haemangioma			1 ×	

[a] Performed with the old urological device

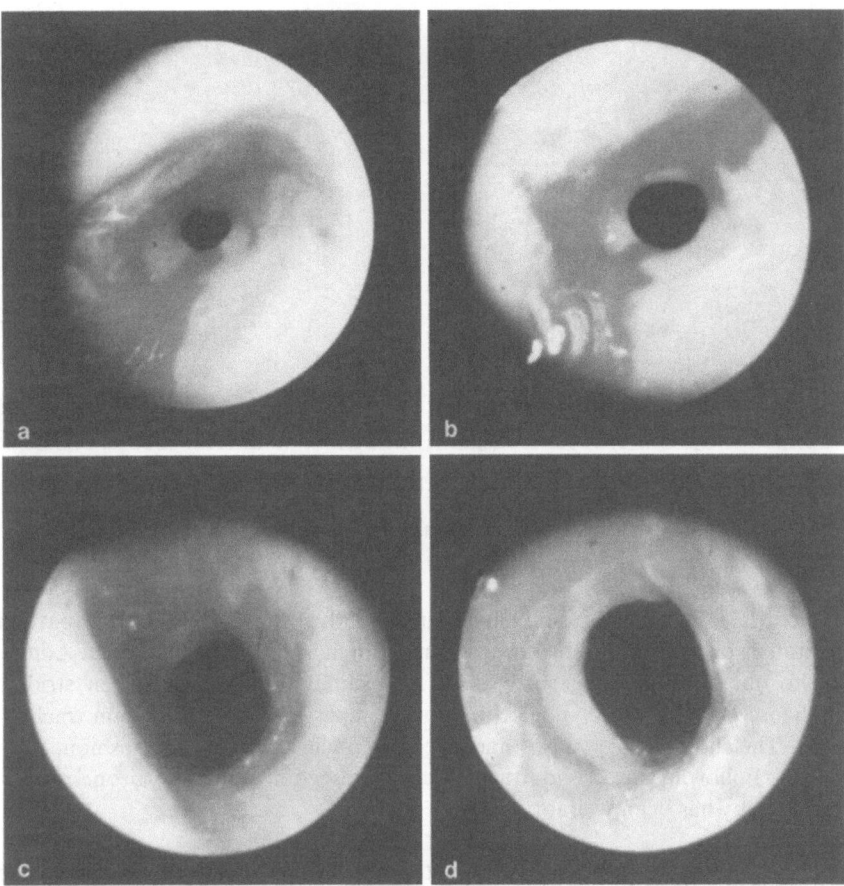

Fig. 4a–d. Case 3. **a** endoscopic picture following several dilatations, **b** after 1 week, **c** after 4 months, **d** after 1 year

Case 3. Male, 1 year (Figs. 3c, d and 4a–d). Emergency intubation for encephalitis with a large No. 5 endotracheal tube. Thereafter intubated patient transferred to our hospital. Respiratory situation necessitated long-term intubation over 12 days. A tracheostomy was carried out on the 13th day for mucosal maceration of the larynx and trachea and for long-term ventilation. Nonetheless, the patient developed an extreme, short-range subglottic stenosis with a residual lumen of 1 mm. Bougienage was started 6 weeks after admission (Figs. 3c and 4a). After 23 dilatations during the following 4 months the child was decannulated (Fig. 4c). However, 20 further dilatations became necessary in the following year to keep the stenosis patent (Fig. 4d). After 2 years, follow-up revealed restenosis which was removed with the resectoscope. Today, 7 years after onset of the disease, the child is well and without signs of restenosis.

5 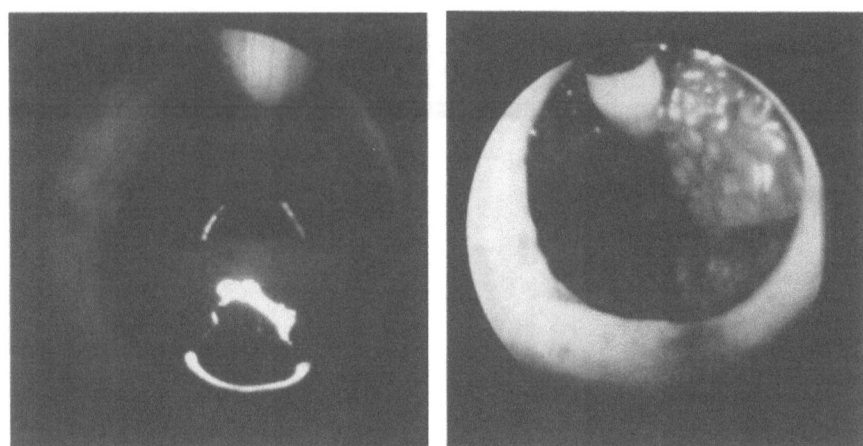 6

Fig. 5. Case 6. Positioning of the resection sling beyond the membrane

Fig. 6. Case 19. Viral papilloma; positioning of the resection sling beyond the papilloma

Case 6. Male, 3 years (Fig. 5). Delivery in the 35th gestational week, post-partum respiratory distress syndrome necessitating artificial ventilation for 9 days. Admission to our hospital at age of 3 years for examination of a persistent stridor. Tracheoscopy revealed a subglottic stenosis impassable with the 3-mm tracheoscope. The short-range stenosis narrowed the trachea in a sail-like fashion, from the left. Following three endotracheal electroresections under cortisone protection, the boy has been well for 2 years.

Case 19. Female, 2 years (Fig. 6). First appearance of viral condylomas in the larynx at the age of 1 year. Repeated laser removals of the condylomas in another hospital. Simultaneous interferon therapy could not overcome recurrences. Treatment was stopped after 1 year because of lack of success. Admission to our hospital at the age of 2 years in a state of serious respiratory insufficiency necessitating immediate tracheostomy (Fig. 6). We tried to control the condylomas which extended down to the main bronchi by three laser applications, without success. In fact there was progression of the condylomas so we proceeded with the resectoscope. Within 1 year, 31 electroresections were carried out, accompanied for the last 6 months by interferon treatment of increasing dosage up to 200000 IU/kg. Depending on the site and extent of the condylomas, electroresections were performed either via tracheostomy or transorally. During the final weeks of treatment we observed for the first time a marked improvement over longer intervals, particularly where cauterization was additionally employed. We lost touch with the child for follow-up since the family emigrated to the United States in April 1987.

Results

It can be seen from Table 1 that, in contrast to bougienage, endoscopic electroresection was rarely employed before 1985. Since the resection device was improved in 1985, electroresection is frequently performed, whereas dilatation treatment is practically obsolete. Despite initially successful bougienage which, however, had to be carried out frequently (43 times), electroresection with the new device finally had to be performed after 2 years in case 3. The device can be favourably and easily applied in the development of granulation tissue at the tracheostomy and, above all, at the anterior tracheal wall.

Discussion

Endotracheal electroresection can be performed with the smallest urological resection device [6]; cases 1, 3, 4). This device, however, has the drawback that it is too short to reach beyond the subglottic region. Moreover, artificial ventilation cannot be provided since the instrument has no integral airway. However, in contrast to the adult size resectoscope so far available, the new device is considerably thinner with an external diameter of 3.5 mm together with the ventilation tube, and is thus suited to severe tracheal stenoses. The mode of treatment depends first on the kind of stenosis and second on its site (see Fig. 2). We differentiate between: (a) short stenoses of the mucosa (membranous stenoses); (b) stenoses including the whole tracheal wall (short or long range); and (c) stenoses caused by destruction or malacia of the cartilaginous skeleton, usually over a longer distance. The procedure is influenced by the site of the stenosis, since distal stenoses can be best treated by transverse resection with end-to-end anastomosis, no matter how long they are [8, 15, 19].

The situation is different in subglottic stenoses. Here the length of the stenosis is decisive for the choice of procedure. Tracheoplasty with complete separation of the stenotic ring and cartilaginous interposition into the posterior tracheal wall (modified according to Hof) seems to be the method of choice in long-distance and severe subglottic stenoses [10]. Operation under 1 year of age, however, carries a high recurrence rate.

Short-distance stenoses, particularly those affecting only the mucosa, can be either dilated, electroresected or treated by laser [1, 3, 6, 12]. Cryotherapy is also recommended [10, 13]. Bougienage is certainly the simplest method [3], but time-consuming (in our patients often more than 50 sessions). As is the case in other methods, bougienage can be successful only in short-distance stenoses. We have no experience with cryotherapy. As far as kind of stenosis is concerned, laser surgery and electroresection have similar success rates. Recurrence rate, which can probably be lowered by adjuvant, high-dose cortisone treatment, is also similar in both methods.

Laser surgery must be carried out under direct view in case difficulties arise in distal tracheal stenoses or stenoses of the main bronchi [6]. Perforations may occur in laser surgery, requiring particularly careful technique. A great advantage of the resectoscope is its relative cheapness. However, some experience is necessary for its application.

The method of electroresection of subglottic stenoses has also been described by other authors [6]. The main problem of the resectoscope for infant urology described by Downing [6] is its relative shortness. Longer instruments, on the other hand, have too large external dimensions. However, especially tracheal stenoses in infancy require very thin devices to pass the stenosis. The possibility of passing the stenosis and resecting it subsequently in a distal—proximal direction is one of the main advantages over laser devices where the stenosis can be coagulated under direct view from a proximal position, but the distal extent of the stenosis cannot be assessed. Our resectoscope achieves precisely that; as soon as the stenosis has been passed, tension on the resectoscope enables full assessment of the stenotic extent and its resection until the situation is clarified.

Resection can be carried out stepwise. However, the instrument must be withdrawn after each step for cleaning since cleaning during resection, as in urethral surgery, is not possible. Large-scale resections (as done in case 19 with endolaryngeal, endotracheal and endobronchial papilloma) can also be carried out, as well as minor resections for biopsy.

Acknowledgements. The resectoscope is produced by Storz, Tuttlingen. This work was supported by the National Bank of Austria, Project Number 1820.

References

1. Berkovits RNP et al (1987) Treatment of congenital cricoid stenosis. Prog Pediatr Surg 21:20–28
2. Cohen RC et al (1985) The successful reconstruction of thoracic tracheal defects with free periosteal grafts. J Pediatr Surg 20 (6):852–858
3. Cotton RT (1984) Pediatric laryngotracheal stenosis. J Pediatr Surg 19 (6):699–704
4. Cotton RT (1985) Prevention and management of laryngeal stenosis in infants and children. J Pediatr Surg 20:845–851
5. Denecke HJ (1962) Die chirurgische Behandlung von Stenosen und Atresien der oberen Luft- und Speisewege. Arch Ohren Nasen Hals Heilkd Z, Hals Nasen Ohrenheilkd 180:461
6. Downing TB, Johnson DG (1979) Excision of subglottic stenosis with the urethral resectoscope. J Pediatr Surg 14:252–257
7. Ganfield RA et al (1982) Pneumothorax with upper airway laser surgery. Anaesthesiology 56:398–399
8. Geißler W et al (1985/86) Formen und Bedeutung der Trachealstenosen. Padiatr Prax 32:487–503
9. Gustafson RA et al (1982) Intercostal muscle and myo-osseous flaps in difficult pediatric thoracic problems. J Pediatr Surg 17:541–545
10. Hof E (1987) Surgical correction of laryngotracheal stenoses in children. Prog Pediatr Surg 21:29–35
11. Klos I, Wurnig P (1984) Zur Abklärung von Stridor und Trachealstenose im Neugeborenenalter und Säuglingsalter. Prax Klin Pneumol 38:295–300
12. Mayer T et al (1980) Experimental subglotic stenosis – histopathologic and bronchoscopic comparison of electrosurgical, cryosurgical and laser resection. J Pediatr Surg 15:944–952

13. Meyer R (1982) Reconstructive surgery of the trachea. Thieme, Stuttgart
14. Minnigerode B et al (1977) Die chirurgische Behandlung von Larynx- und Trachealstenosen nach translaryngealer intratrachealer Dauerintubation im Kindesalter. Z Kinderchir 22:111–120
15. Salzer GM, Hartl H, Wurnig P (1987) Treatment of tracheal stenosis by resection in infancy and early childhood. In: Wurnig P (ed)
16. Strome M et al (1982) Advances in management of laryngeal and subglottic stenosis. J Pediatr Surg 17:591–596
17. Wurnig P, Hopfgartner L (1978) Correlation bronchoskopischer und röntgenologischer Befunde im Kindesalter. Padiatr Fortbildungskurse Prax 46:48–63
18. Wurnig P, Hartl H, Salzer GM, Frisch H (1985) Trachealresektionen bei Säuglingen und Kleinkindern. Prax Klin Pneumol 39:588–589
19. Wurnig P, Klos I, Geißler W (1986) Die Bougierungsbehandlung bei Trachealstenosen. Report on the Kinderchirurgisch-kinderanästhesiologisch-intensivmedizinisches Symposium der Südwestdeutschen Tagung für Kinderheilkunde. Saarbrücken

Experimental Studies on Caustic Burns of the Stomach by Aggressive Chemicals

J. Wit, L. Noack, K. Gdanietz, and K. Vorpahl

Summary

The treatment of caustic burns of the stomach in childhood by acids, alkalis and especially soldering fluids has remained without any clear concept so far. Surgical treatment consists of therapy of acute complications or late sequelae. Early endoscopy enables one to decide between conservative treatment and early laparotomy. Animal experiments were performed in albino rats for the development of a therapeutic concept. Because of its amphoteric and aggressive nature, soldering fluid zinc dissolved in 33–$50 M$ saline) was used as the caustic substance. Clear demarcation and tissue changes can be recognized after 6–8 h, at the earliest. Laparotomy aiming at protective plication or atypical gastric resection should be performed at that time, if endoscopy reveals a third-degree caustic burn of the stomach.

Zusammenfassung

Die Behandlung von Verätzungen des kindlichen Magens mit Säuren, Laugen und insbesondere durch Lötwasser erfolgte bisher ohne ein klares Therapiekonzept. Chirurgisch wurden akute Komplikationen oder Spätfolgen behandelt. Durch die Frühendoskopie ist eine Entscheidung zwischen konservativem Vorgehen und der Notwendigkeit der Frühlaparotomie möglich. Zur Erarbeitung eines Therapiekonzepts führten die Autoren tierexperimentelle Untersuchungen an Albinoratten durch. Als Verätzungsmittel wurde wegen seines amphoteren Charakters und seiner besonderen Aggressivität Lötwasser (gelöstes Zink in 33–50 n Salzsäure) verwendet. Eine ausreichende Demarkierung und Gewebsveränderung ist frühestens nach 6–8 h endoskopisch zu erkennen. Die Laparotomie mit dem Ziel einer protektiven Plikatur oder einer atypischen Magenresektion des verätzten Bezirks ist zu diesem Zeitpunkt anzustreben, wenn der endoskopische Befund eine drittgradige Verätzung vermuten läßt.

Résumé

Le traitement des brûlures caustiques de l'estomac des enfants par acides, bases et particulièrement par eau à souder ne repose à l'heure actuelle sur aucune conception thérapeutique précise. La chirurgie restait la seule arme en cas de complications aigües ou ultérieures. Grâce à l'endoscopie précoce, la décision entre un traitement conservateur et une laparotomie précoce peut être envisagée. Afin de mettre au point un protocole thérapeutique, notre expérimentation et nos recherches ont porté sur des rats albinos. Comme substance caustique, nous avons utilisé une solution d'étain dilué dans de l'acide chlorhydrique de 33 à 50 degrés, du fait du caractère amphotère de la substance et de sa causticité. La lésion caustique apparat donc très nettement à l'endoscopie dès les 6 à 8 premières heures. Une laparotomie soit à visée de création d'un pli protecteur, soit à visée de résection d'une partie de l'estomac, doit alors être effectuée, si l'exploration endoscopique met en évidence une lésion du 3ème degré.

Paediatric Surgical Clinic and Outpatients Clinic, Klinikum Berlin-Buch, DDR-1115 Berlin-Buch, German Democratic Republic

Progress in Pediatric Surgery, Vol. 25
Angerpointner (Ed.)
© Springer-Verlag Berlin Heidelberg 1990

Patients and Method

Gastric burns of the major curvature of the stomach were produced by instillation of 0.15 ml soldering fluid via a gastric tube in Wistar rats weighing 200–300 g, under ether anaesthesia. Surgery was performed following intraperitoneal application of pentobarbital. Metallic zinc occupies group IIB of the periodic table and is amphoteric. Zinc is present as an aquo complex in the soldering fluid.

$$H_2O \quad H_2O$$
$$\backslash / $$
$$Zn-Zn(OH)_2$$

Zincates are produced in acidic environments and two reaction mechanisms ensue, with production of heat

$$Zn^{2+} + 6H_2O \rightarrow [Zn\,H_2O_6]^{2-}$$

$$Zn^{2+} + 3Zn(OH)_2 \rightarrow \left[Zn\left(Zn{<}^{OH}_{OH}\right)_3\right]^{2-}$$

These anions form complexes with proteins. Together with zinc, the NH_4Cl which is present in small amounts creates zinc ammonium chloride

$$(NH_4)_2[ZnCl_4]$$

Soldering fluid shows reactions which are different from those of pure acids or alkalis.

Experimental Protocol

The following questions needed to be clarified:

1. Extent of gastric damage in relation to duration of influence
2. Relation of mucosal changes to changes of the serosa
3. Relation of macroscopic to microscopic changes of the gastric wall
4. Determination of the optimal time of operation
5. When is plication and when is gastric resection indicated?

Since the histological structure and functional nature of the rat stomach is similar to that of the human, rats seemed best suited for our experiments.

Results and Discussion

Between 1971 and 1987, 23 children were admitted to our hospital (Berlin-Buch) for ingestion of soldering fluid; of these children, 7 required surgery. It was shown that the postoperative course following primary surgery was uneventful in four children with endoscopically diagnosed third-degree caustic burns of the stomach. Protective plications of the gastric wall over the affected region or atypical gastric resections were carried out. Children with third-degree caustic burns who were primarily treated conservatively had to undergo surgery later on for sequelae of the burns, i.e. haemorrhage, perforation, gastrocolic fistula, bowel obstruction. Considerable shrinkage of the stomach could be observed, as described by other authors [2, 4, 6]. There is a considerable difference in the clinical courses of third-degree caustic burns of the stomach following primarily conservative or surgical procedures. The pH-dependent mode of action of soldering fluid explains the relative intactness of oesophagus and duodenum. The stomach is the primary target. In order to avoid severe complications which may be difficult to control, or late sequelae (gastric shrinkage, fistulization), primary surgical treatment of third-degree caustic burns of the stomach is recommended [1, 3, 5].

Therapeutic recommendations in the literature for adults range from primarily conservative treatment to immediate gastrectomy. Experimental studies with the aim of organ-preserving treatment in childhood have not been performed so far. We obtained the following results:

1. Macroscopic demarcation of the affected region can be expected 4–6 h after ingestion, at the earliest. Thus laparotomy should not be carried out before this. However, later laparotomy carries the risk of early perforation.
2. Protective plication or atypical, organ-preserving gastric resection come into consideration as surgical methods.
3. Even in third-degree caustic burns (absent serosal gloss) plication prevents perforation and controls late sequelae. This procedure might be best employed in extended gastric burns.
4. In minor burns, however, we prefer atypical resection. Atomic spectrometry has shown that resection must be carried out far into healthy tissue in these instances, since zinc can be detected even in seemingly healthy surrounding tissue. Otherwise, gastric shrinkage could result.
5. In all our experiments, we found the pylorus tightly closed by reflex pylorospasm. Therefore, duodenum and small intestine were never affected.
6. Reparative processes were finished within 4 weeks.

The early protective operation after 4–6 h with initial endoscopy is far superior to late surgery for complications. Close cooperation of endoscopists, paediatricians and paediatric surgeons is therefore essential.

References

1. Brugsch H, Klimmer OR (1966) Vergiftungen im Kindesalter. Enke, Stuttgart
2. Gögler H, Wolf S, Ibse K, Bücher ES (1988) Verätzungen des oberen Gastrointesinaltraktes bei Erwachsenen. Zentralbl Chir 113:345–350
3. Jung FJ, Gdanietz K (1978) Ingestionsunfälle durch Lötwasser im Kindesalter. Kinderaertzl Prax 46:184–189
4. Möschlin S (1972) Klinik und Therapie der Vergiftungen. Thieme, Stuttgart
5. Mühlendal KE, Krienke ES (1979/80) Vergiftungen im Kindesalter – Gefahren der Obertherapie bei Kindern. Paediatr Prax 22:607–611
6. Rehbein F, Reismann B (1965) Speiseröhren- und Magenverätzungen bei Kindern. Langenbecks Arch Klin Chir 311:100–113

Intraperitoneal Application of Fibrinogen Gluing in the Rat for Adhesions Prophylaxis

J. L. Koltai and A. Gerhard

Summary

The suitability of fibrinogen gluing for prophylaxis of intraperitoneal adhesions was investigated experimentally. Small bowel slings, traumatized previously, were covered by a layer of fibrinogen 2–3 mm thick to see whether formation of adhesions could be prevented. In the experiments 50 rats of both sexes were observed over 21 days. Following mechanical traumatization of the terminal ileum the visceral peritoneum was coated with fibronogen, whereas animals of the control group did not receive fibrinogen coating.

Macroscopic and microscopic findings after 1, 3, 7, 14 and 21 days yielded the following results:

1. Fibrinogen dissolution and resorption occurred for 3–14 days following operation.
2. On autopsy, all animals of the control group showed massive, extended adhesions; two of the controls died on the 6th postoperative day from peritonitis.
3. None of the treated animals exhibited extended adhesions.
4. Histological examinations revealed regeneration of the injured serosa and healing of the bowel wall below the fibrinogen coating.
5. Fibrinogen applied to intact peritoneal serosa (without injury) is entirely resorbed without formation of adhesions.

Zusammenfassung

Die Eignung von Fibrinkleber zur Prophylaxe von intraperitonealen Adhäsionen wurde tierexperimentell überprüft. Dabei wurde versucht, die zuvor traumatisierten Dünndarmschlingen mit einer schützenden, 2–3 mm dicken Lage von Fibrin zu überziehen und damit eine Adhäsionsbildung zu verhindern. In den Experimenten wurden hierzu 50 Ratten beiderlei Geschlechts im Verlauf von 21 Tagen beobachtet. Nach mechanischer Traumatisierung des terminalen Ileums wurde Fibrinkleber auf das viszerale Peritoneum aufgebracht. In einer Kontrollgruppe erhielten die Tiere keine Behandlung mit Fibrinkleber.

Die makroskopischen und mikroskopischen Befunde nach 1, 3, 7, 14 und 21 Tagen zeigten, daß

1) die Auflösung und Resorption des Fibrins in einem Zeitraum von 3–14 Tagen nach der Operation stattfand;
2) von den Kontrolltieren 2 am 6. postoperativen Tag vorzeitig an einer massiven Peritonitis verstarben und alle Kontrolltiere bei der Obduktion massive flächenhafte Verwachsungen zeigten;
3) in keinem Fall der therapeutischen Gruppe flächenhafte Verwachsungen beobachtet werden konnten;

Paediatric Surgical Clinic, Johannes Gutenberg University, Langenbeck Strasse 1, D-6500 Mainz, Federal Republic of Germany

Progress in Pediatric Surgery, Vol. 25
Angerpointner (Ed.)
© Springer-Verlag Berlin Heidelberg 1990

4) die histologischen Untersuchungen eine Regeneration der verletzten Darmserosa und eine Abheilung der verletzten Darmwandschichten unter dem Fibrinbelag aufwiesen;

5. Fibrinkleber auf intakter peritonealer Serosa (ohne Traumatisierung) restlos absorbiert wurde und eine Adhäsionsbildung nicht zustande kam.

Résumé

L'expérience animale a confirmé l'efficacité d'une colle à base de fibrine dans la prophylaxie des brides intrapéritonéales. A cet effet, on a essayé d'entourer de fibrine sur une épaisseur de 2 à 3 mm, des anses intestinales grêles traumatisées et ceci afin de limiter le phénomène de brides. Pour ce faire, 50 rats des deux sexes ont été mis en observation pendant 21 jours. Après leur avoir entraîné mécaniquement une irritation iléale, cette colle à la fibrine fut appliquée sur le péritoine. Le groupe témoin, lui, ne reçut pas de colle.

Les lésions macroscopiques et microscopiques retrouvées aux 1er, 3ème, 7ème, 14ème et 21ème jours montraient:

1) la disparition et la résorption de la fibrine entre le 3ème et le 14ème jour après l'opération,
2) deux des animaux témoins étaient morts au 6ème jour et tous les autres avaient montré, à la vérification, d'importantes adhérences étendues;
3) qu'e aucun cas, un tel phénomène n'avait été observé chez les animaux traités;
4) que l'étude histologique montrait une régénération de la séreuse lésée et une récupération de la muqueuse recouverte par la fibrine et le fait que
5) la colle à la fibrine déposée sur une séreuse intacte avait été totalement résorbée sans laisser aucune trace d'adhésion

Introduction

The use of fibrinogen gluing has become an established part of postoperative treatment for the last 10 years. Despite many pros and cons more and more new fields of application have emerged. Intraperitoneally, fibrinogen gluing is mainly used for organ-preserving operations in liver or splenic rupture or for adjuvant protection of endangered intestinal anastomoses [3, 5, 22, 27, 28]. Most authors, however, emphasize that fibrinogen gluing must not be used as a substitute for conventional operative techniques.

Although the role and biochemical pathways of physiological fibrinogen in the formation of intraperitoneal adhesions were defined by Milligan and Raftery [24] in 1974, experimental studies on the effects of fibrinogen gluing on adhesions have not been carried out until recently.

In 1984 Lindenberg and Lauritzen [19] produced ischaemic defects at the parietal peritoneum and sealed the defects by fibrinogen gluing after primary suture. Based on the pathogenesis of adhesion formation, they expected an adhesion-promoting effect. However, they found a preventative effect instead. Further experiments have shown that the concentration of the fibrinolysis inhibitor aprotinin, usually embodied in fibrinogen glue, did not show any effect, whereas the amount of applied fibrinogen glue played a major role.

Hjortrup et al. [16] reported similar results: they observed a lesser trend to formation of adhesions in a comparative study on the strength of sutured and glued anastomoses when fibrinogen glue was used additionally. Brands et al. [6] secured intestinal anastomoses with three or four marginal sutures and modified the mesenteric plication according to Childs-Philipps [7] with fibrinogen gluing.

In our experimental work we tried to find answers to two questions:

1. What happens to fibrinogen glue applied to intact peritoneum?
2. Is there indeed a possibility of adhesion prophylaxis in severe peritoneal defects by means of application of a thick fibrinogen layer?

Patients and Method

For the experiments 50 rats of both sexes were used, anaesthetized with combined ether–ketamine. Anaesthesia was induced by ether inhalation and maintained by intraperitoneal application (4–6 mg/kg) of ketamine. A left-sided paramedian laparotomy was carried out. The lowest three slings of the terminal ileum were chosen for later application of fibrinogen glue to give a clearly defined anatomical region. The fibrinogen glue Tissucol was sprayed on the visceral peritoneum by means of a pressure set (Tissomat-Immuno; sterile driving gas; pressure 2–3 bar) so that the thin spraying catheter provided an optimal mixture of the gluing components.

In the control group A ($n = 3$) about 10 cm of the terminal ileum was positioned side by side, fixed by fibrinogen coating and reduced to the abdominal cavity (Fig. 1). The muscle-peritoneal layer was closed by a running, 4–0 catgut suture. The skin was closed by a running monofilament nonabsorbable suture. In the remaining animals the terminal ileum was traumatized by means of a surgical forceps (Fig. 2). Thereafter, the intestinal surface was coated with fibrinogen glue in the manner already mentioned. The animals of control group B were operated

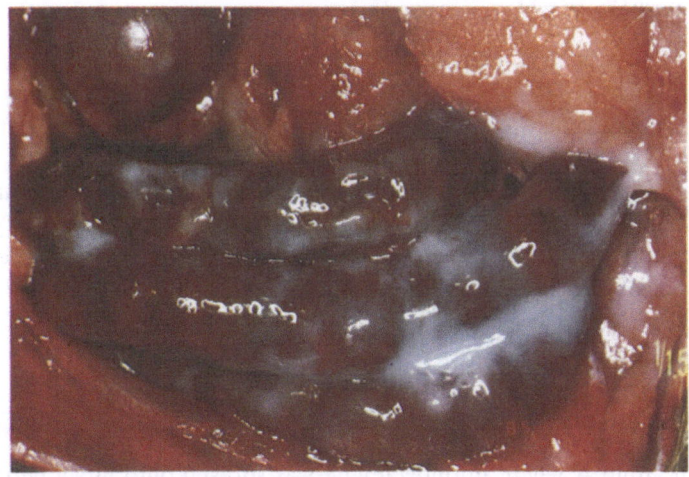

Fig. 1. Whitish gelatinous coating on the terminal ileum following fibrinogen application

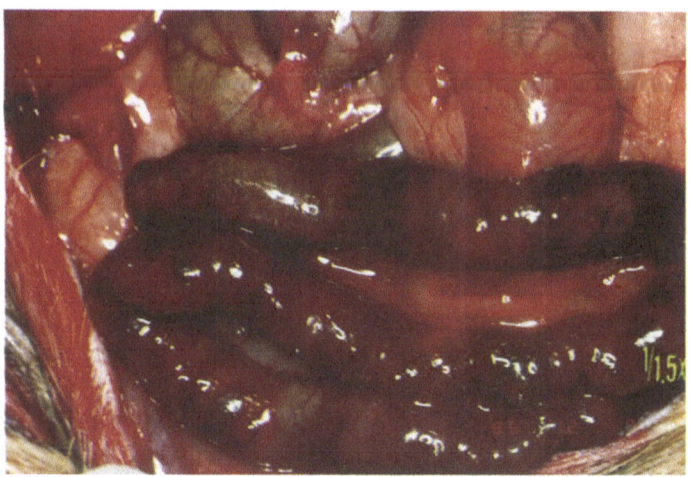

Fig. 2. Terminal ileum following traumatization

Table 1. Treatment and control groups in the study

Group		Follow-up time (days)	Treatment	
			Fibrinogen glue	Bowel injury
Control A	$(n = 3)$	1	+	−
Control B	$(n = 7)$	6 $(n = 2)$ 10 $(n = 4)$ 21 $(n = 1)$	−	+
Group I	$(n = 5)$	1	+	+
Group II	$(n = 9)$	3	+	+
Group III	$(n = 9)$	7	+	+
Group IV	$(n = 8)$	14	+	+
Group V	$(n = 9)$	21	+	+

on in the same way with traumatization of the terminal ileum, but without fibrinogen coating.

The animals of the different groups were killed 1, 3, 7, 14 and 21 days postoperatively and investigated macroscopically and microscopically (Table 1). The traumatized terminal ileum was excised in toto, fixed in 4% formaldehyde, stained with haematoxylin-eosin and van Gieson's and evaluated histologically.

Results

Macroscopic Findings

In group A where fibrinogen glue was sprayed onto intact peritoneum its complete resorption occurred within 24 h. There were no adhesions and bowel motility was unimpaired. In the control group B where the bowel slings were traumatized, but no fibrinogen glue was applied, two animals died on the 6th post-operative day from massive peritonitis. Four animals exhibited several adhesion cords and extended adhesions on the 10th postoperative day (Fig. 3). One animal killed on the 21st day showed four strong adhesion cords.

It could be shown that in the other animals the fibrinogen glue remained unchanged for 1–4 days as a white, gelatinous coating so that the bowel slings persisted in their adapted position below the fibrinogen layer (Figs. 4 and 5). After

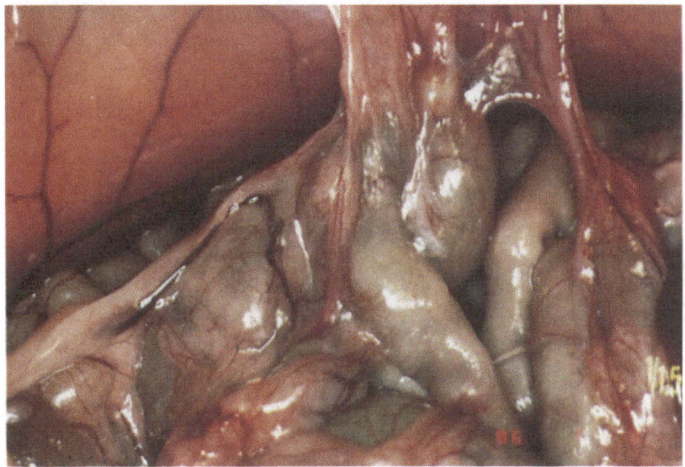

Fig. 3. Control group B (no fibrinogen glue, bowel injury): extended adhesions and adhesion cords after 10 days

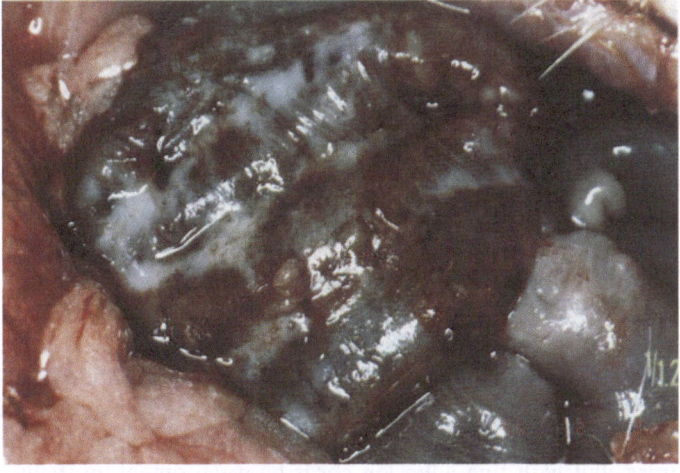

Fig. 4. Persistent fibrinogen coating at the visceral peritoneum after 24 h

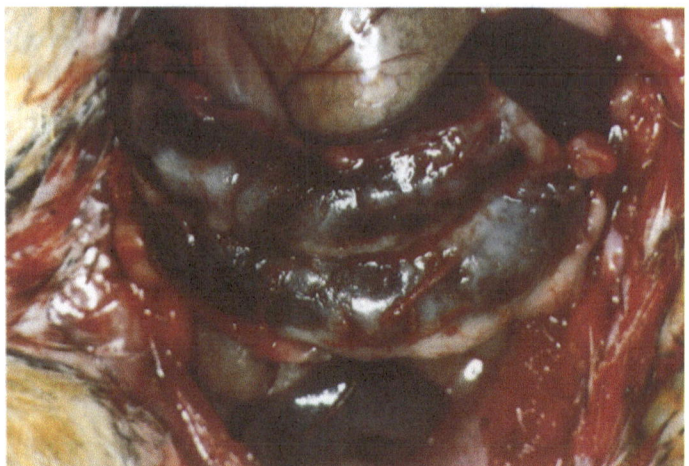

Fig. 5. Partial fibrinogen resorption after 3 days

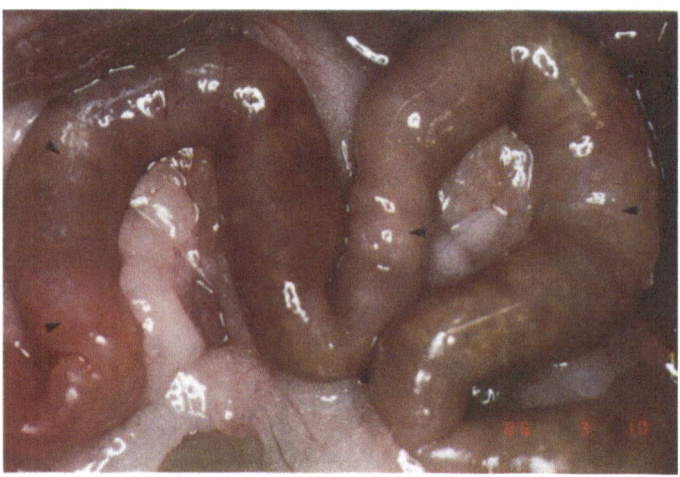

Fig. 6. Complete fibrinogen resorption, free bowel motility and healing of the serosa after 21 days. *Arrowheads* show former perforations of the bowel wall

7 days the fibrinogen glue was entirely resorbed with free motility of the bowel slings in four of nine animals. In the other five cases adhesive fibrinogen remnants were still present.

In the next group of eight animals complete resorption of fibrinogen could be shown in all cases after 14 days. Four animals had free motility of the bowel slings and no adhesions. The four remaining cases showed healing of the traumatized serosa, but with fine adhesion cords between omentum, bowels and abdominal wall.

Complete resorption of fibrinogen was demonstrated after 21 days in all nine animals of the last group. Seven animals did not present with adhesions and the bowel surface was entirely intact. Only some whitish spots indicated the former injuries (Fig. 6). Only two animals presented in the marginal area with one adhesion cord each.

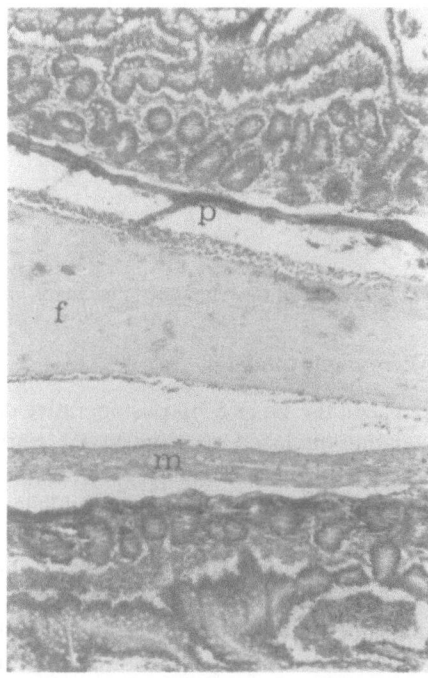

Fig. 7. Persistent fibrinogen coating *(f)* between bowel slings at a perforation point *(p):* muscularis *(m)* interrupted. H & E

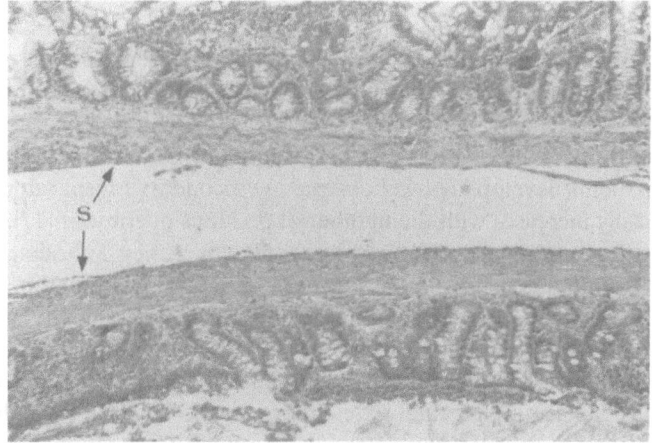

Fig. 8. Serosal regeneration *(s)* after 14 days; H & E

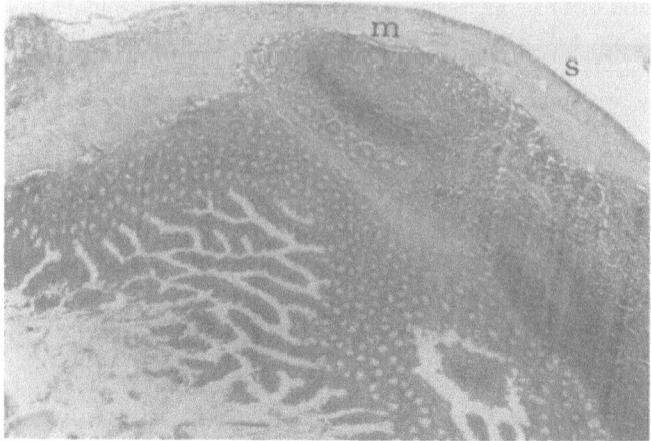

Fig. 9. Healing of the diminished muscularis *(m)* and serosa *(s)* at the perforation point. H & E

Microscopic Findings

Between the 1st and 3rd postoperative days, haematoxylin-eosin and van Gieson's staining disclosed well-preserved fibrinogen glue between the bowel slings (Fig. 7). In the marginal area an aggregation of polymorphonuclear leucocytes, some macrophages and eosinophil leucocytes could be observed.

Progressive decrease of the thickness of the fibrinogen layer ensued from the 3rd postoperative day on. By the 7th, or at the latest the 14th postoperative day, the fibrinogen between the bowel slings had entirely vanished histologically. At the same time the bowel serosa was completely regenerated (Fig. 8). Below the healed serosa, scarry infiltrations appeared within the whitish spots already mentioned, where the bowel wall had been perforated (Fig. 9).

Discussion

Formation of adhesions is a frequently observed reaction of the human body to laparotomy [1, 12]. Ellis [10, 11], for instance, reported that 67% of all patients who had undergone a laparotomy developed adhesions. Meier et al. [23], Festen [13] and Wilkins and Spitz [31] found out that 10%–30% of paediatric surgical patients developed bowel obstruction secondary to laparotomy. This rate dramatically increases with the number of previous operations [17]. Mere detachment of adhesions as necessary, however, only effects new adhesions of the same extent.

One aspect of the pathogenesis of adhesion formation is the genesis of the fibrin network with counteracting fibrinolytic activity; regeneration of the peritoneum and the subserosal tissue is the other aspect. Adhesions develop if decomposition of fibrinogen by normal fibrinolytic activity of the mesothelial cells takes place earlier than regeneration of the bowel serosa, thus affecting the formation of collagen and, later, of adhesions by activation of connective tissue macrophages and fibroblasts [10, 11, 15, 18, 24].

Numerous methods have been evaluated experimentally and clinically in order to influence these processes [21]. For this purpose various substances, such as corticosteroids [14], the fibrinolysis inhibitor aprotinin [26, 32], fibrinolytic substances [2, 23] and fibroblast proliferation inhibitors [8, 14] have been employed. None of these methods, however, found its way into practice, since clinical application could not prevent the formation of adhesions.

A new approach was shown by Lindenberg et al. [19, 20] by intraperitoneal application of fibrinogen gluing. One would expect an increased creation of adhesions by spreading fibrinogen onto the peritoneum. However, the authors found that the development of adhesions by peritoneal ischaemic defects could be prevented. This effect could be amplified by increasing the thickness of the fibrinogen layer. Decomposition and resorption of the fibrinogen which take place for 3–7 days postoperatively (as shown in the work reported here) is organized by neutrophil granulocytes and macrophages [9]. Mesothelial repair starts within 2–3 days [26] and is completed within 5 days at the peritoneum. We were thus able to show in our experiments that application of fibrinogen glue in a layer of 2–3 mm may reinforce the protective function of the remaining fibrinogen until regeneration of the mesothelium, i.e. the bowel serosa, is completed. Our histological findings impressively indicated the regeneration of the serosa and the bowel wall while the protective fibrinogen layer was slowly decomposed and resorbed by fibrinolysis.

A single application of fibrinogen glue does not induce an immunological response. Comparison of rat fibrinogen with human fibrinogen did not reveal significant differences as far as preventative effects were concerned [19, 20]. Corresponding application in adults would require huge amounts of fibrinogen glue, probably restricting routine use for economic reasons. Nevertheless, this therapeutic concept provides a toehold for the solution of problems with adhesions following laparotomies. So far our clinical experience with the use of fibrinogen gluing in bowel obstruction in infancy corresponds well with the positive results in gynaecological patients reported by Westen [30], where fertility problems secondary to massive adhesions in the lower abdomen could be positively influenced by adhesiolysis and use of fibrinogen gluing.

References

1. Alameddine A (1979) Peritoneal adhesions: where do we stand? Md Med J 28:48–49
2. Ascherl R, Wriedt-Lübbe I, Rothe M, Birk M, Wendt P, Petrowitz O, Stemberger A, Blümel G (1983) Prophylaxis of intraperitoneal adhesions with a fibrinolytic agent. Experimental studies of the efficacy and the possible effect on wound healing. Med Welt 34:410–415
3. Blocker SH, Ternberg JL (1986) Traumatic liver laceration in newborn. Repair with fibrin glue. J Pediatr Surg 21:369–371
4. Braenstedt S, Olson PS (1980) Effect of defibrinogenation on wound strength and collagen formation. A study in rabbits. Acta Chir Scand 146:483–486
5. Brands W, Beck M, Raute-Kreinsen U (1981) Gewebeklebung der rupturierten Milz mit hochkonzentriertem Fibrinogen. Z Kinderchir 32:1–8
6. Brands W, Joppich I, Lochbühler H (1982) Use of highly concentrated human fibrinogen in pediatric surgery. A new therapeutic principle. Z Kinderchir 35:159–162

7. Childs W, Philipps (1960) Experience with intestinal plication and a proposed modification. Ann Surg 152:258–265
8. Dargenio R (1986) Pharmacological prevention of postoperative adhesions experimentally induced in the rat. Acta Eur Fertil 17:267–272
9. Dinges HP, Redl H, Kuderna H, Matras H (1979) Histologie nach Fibrinklebung. Dtsch Z Mund Kiefer Gesichts Chir 3:29–31
10. Ellis H (1980) Internal overhealing: the problem of peritoneal adhesions. World J Surg 4:303–306
11. Ellis H (1982) The causes and prevention of intestinal adhesions. Br J Surg 69:241–243
12. Fedor E, Miko I, Nagy T (1983) The role of ischemia in the formation of postoperative intra-abdominal adhesions. Acta Chir Hung 24:3–8
13. Festen H (1982) Postoperative small bowel obstruction in infants and children. Ann Surg 196:580–583
14. Granat M (1983) Reduction of peritoneal adhesion by colchicine. A comparative study in the rat. Fertil Steril 40:369–372
15. Hedelin H, Johansson S, Peterson HI, Teger-Nilsson A-c, Pettersson S (1982) Influence of fibrin clots on development of granulation tissue in preformed cavities. Surg Gynaecol Obstet 154:521–525
16. Hjortrup A, Nordkild PJ, Kiaergaard J, Sjontroft E, Olesen HP (1986) Fibrin adhesives versus sutured anastomosis. A comparative intraindividual study in the small intestine of pigs. Br J Surg 73:760–761
17. Janik JS (1981) An assessment of the surgical treatment of adhesive small bowel obstruction in infants and children. J Pediat Surg 16:225–235
18. Kapur BML, Kumar R, Chopra P (1984) Pathogenesis of reformation of intraperitoneal adhesions in albino rats. Indian J Med Res 79:244–249
19. Lindenberg S, Lauritsen JG (1984) Prevention of peritoneal adhesion formation by fibrin sealant. An experimental study in rats. Ann Chir Gynaecol (Helsinki) 73:11–13
20. Lindenberg S, Steentoft P, Sorensen SS, Olesen HP (1985) Studies on prevention of intra-abdominal adhesion formation by fibrin sealant. An experimental study in rats. Acta Chir Scand 151:525–527
21. Marais C, Sasse V, McComb P, Gomel V (1985) A comparative study on the suppression of peritoneal adhesion formation in the rat. Acta Eur Fertil 16:267–271
22. Marczell A, Efferdinger F, Spoula H, Stierer M (1979) Anwendungsbereiche des Fibrinklebers in der Abdominalchirurgie. Acta Chir Austr 11:137–141
23. Meier H, Dietl KH, Willital GH (1985) Erste klinische Ergebnisse der intraoperativen Adhäsionsprophylaxe bei Kindern. Langenbecks Arch Chir 366:191–193
24. Milligan GW, Raftery AT (1974) Observation on the pathogenesis of peritoneal adhesions. A light and electron microscopical study. Br J Surg 61:274–280
25. Pflugler H, Redl H (1982) Abbau von Fibrinkleber in vivo und in vitro (Versuche an der Ratte). Z Urol Nephrol 75:25–30
26. Raftery AT (1979) Noxythiolin (Noxyflex), aprotinin (Trasylol) and peritoneal adhesion formation. An experimental study in the rat. Br J Surg 66:654–656
27. Roth H, Daum R, Bolkenius M (1982) Partielle Milzresektion mit Fibrinklebung – Eine Alternative zur Splenektomie und Autotransplantation. Z Kinderchir 35:153–156
28. Scheele J (1984) Fibrinklebung. Springer, Berlin Heidelberg New York Tokyo
29. Vemer HM, Rolland R (1984) Prevention of adhesion formation in the abdomen and microsurgical methods for the treatment of infertility due to adhesions. Ned. Tijdschr Geneeskd 128:2180–2183
30. Westen A (1987) Erste Erfahrungen über Anwendung des Fibrinklebers bei Peritonealdefekten im kleinen Becken. In: Kubli F, Schmidt W, Gauwerky J (eds) Fibrinklebung in der Frauenheilkunde und Geburtshilfe. Springer, Berlin Heidelberg New York, pp 135–139
31. Wilkins B, Spitz L (1986) Incidence of postoperative adhesion obstruction following neonatal laparotomy. Br J Surg 73:762–764
32. Young HL, Wheeler MH, Morse D (1981) The effect of intravenous aprotinin (Trasylol) on intraperitoneal adhesion formation in the rat. Br J Surg 68:59–60

Surgical Techniques in Short Bowel Syndrome

K. L. Waag and K. Heller

Summary

An operation according to Bianchi in a 2-year-old girl is described and indications as well as technical procedure are discussed. The girl was born with a gastroschisis. There was a jejunal perforation 10 cm below the ligament of Treitz caused by a volvulus. Only 20 cm of the jejunum remained. Moreover, only the left part of the colon was present. Total parenteral nutrition for 2 years was necessary. The principle of the operation is based on a longitudinal division of the remaining bowel and a creation of two separate bowel tubes out of the divided bowel halves, thus effecting an isoperistaltic serial connection by means of two anastomoses. This is technically possible since each half of the bowel wall has its own blood supply. The vessels originating from the mesenterium branch off before they reach the bowel wall so that the mesenteric dissection line can be anastomosed longitudinally with the antimesenteric border. This results in doubling of the bowel length, narrowing of the preoperatively dilated bowel diameter, closer contact of bowel contents with the mucosa, prolonged transit time and a *Bacteroides* colonization which is reduced by more effective peristalsis. Indications, time of operation and our own experiences are discussed and three cases are described. All children are alive and show marked improvement in nutrition.

Zusammenfassung

Am Beispiel der Erfahrungen bei einem 2jährigen Mädchen wird die Operation nach Bianchi beschrieben; Indikationen sowie technisches Vorgehen werden diskutiert. Das Mädchen war mit einer Gastroschisis geboren worden. Es bestand eine Jejunumperforation 10 cm unterhalb des Treitz-Bandes, verursacht durch einen Volvulus, so daß nur 20 cm Restjejunum blieben. Darüber hinaus war nur die linke Hälfte des Kolons angelegt. Eine totale parenterale Ernährung über 2 Jahre war erforderlich.

Das Prinzip der Operation besteht in der Längsspaltung des Restdarmes und der Umformung dieser 2 Darmhälften in 2 separate Röhren, die durch Anastomosen isoperistaltisch hintereinander geschaltet werden. Die Gefäße teilen sich, vom Mesenterium kommend, bereits vor der Darmwand mesenterialseits auf, so daß der mesenteriale Darmschnittrand mit dem antimesenterialen Rand längs anastomosiert werden kann. Daraus resultiert eine Verdoppelung der Darmlänge, eine Verkleinerung des präoperativ meist dilatierten Darmabschnitts, ein besserer Speisebreikontakt mit der Mukosa, eine verlängerte Transitzeit und eine durch effektivere Peristaltik verminderte Bacteroidesbesiedelung.

Es wird auf die Indikation und den Operationszeitpunkt bzw. auf die eigenen Erfahrungen eingegangen und 3 Kasuistiken werden diskutiert. Alle Kinder überlebten und haben bei der oralen Nahrungsaufnahme entscheidende Fortschritte gemacht.

Division of Paediatric Surgery, Zentrum der Chirurgie, Johann Wolfang Goethe University, Theodor-Stern-Kai 7, D-6000 Frankfurt am Main, Federal Republic of Germany

Progress in Pediatric Surgery, Vol. 25
Angerpointner (Ed.)
© Springer-Verlag Berlin Heidelberg 1990

Résumé

A titre de démonstration, nous discutons l'opération d'après Bianchi, réalisée sur une fillette de 2 ans. Elle présentait de naissance une laparoschisis. Il y avait une perforation jujénale à 10 cm sous de ligament de Treitz, due à un volvulus, de telle sorte qu'il ne restait que 20 cm de jéjunum. En outre, il n'existait que la partie gauche du colon. Cette fillette a été nourrie pendant 2 ans de façon parentérale exclusive. L'idée opératoire était de faire une incision longitudinale de la partie restante de l'intestin, réalisant ainsi deux moitiés d'anses intestinales qui seront anastomosées en une seule anse. Les vaisseaux d'origine mésentérique bifurqueront avant la paroi intestinale dans le mésentère, de façon à ce qu'ils puissent être anastomosés sur le côté antémésentérial. De cela il résulte un doublement de la longuer de l'intestin, une diminution du calibre intestinal, un meilleur contact entre le bol alimentaire et la muqueuse, un temps de transit intestinal rallongé et un péristaltisme actif, diminuant la stase bactérienne. 3 autres cas ont été discutés et ont permis de fixer le protocole. Tous les enfants survécurent et purent améliorer leur alimentation orale.

Introduction

Every paediatric surgical centre where neonates are operated on is aware of the problem of the short bowel syndrome. Progress in long-term total parenteral nutrition (TPN) and development of long-term implantable catheters, such as the Hickman, Proviac and Infus-a-port devices, have improved the situation so that a longer bowel adaptation time and satisfactory weight gain are possible. However, problems such as catheter sepsis may arise from long-term TPN. A final decision on the fate of those children who are unable to come off long-term TPN may be delayed, but is usually forced by a catheter sepsis. Therefore, the development of techniques for early surgical procedures is mandatory in the short bowel syndrome.

Method

The principle of the operation which was experimentally developed in seven pigs with short bowel syndrome was published by Bianchi of Manchester in 1980 [4]. Total bowel length was 10–30 cm. The remaining bowel is divided longitudinally and the two bowel halves are transformed into two separate tubes which are subsequently connected in series. Longitudinal division becomes possible by the fact that each half of the bowel circumference possesses its own blood supply. The vessels originating from the mesenterium bifurcate before they reach the mesenteric border of the bowel wall, thus providing a space between left and right vascular levels. This space is wide enough to allow longitudinal division of the bowel wall between the bifurcated vessels (Fig. 1). Longitudinal anastomosis is then carried out between the mesenteric and antimesenteric borders of the divided bowel (Figs. 2, 3a, and 3b). Instrumental or manual anastomosis establishes two parallel tubes, each of half the original diameter. A further end-to-end-anastomosis connects these tubes in series isoperistaltically, thus doubling the bowel length (Fig. 4). The remaining proximal and distal openings are anastomosed in the usual manner.

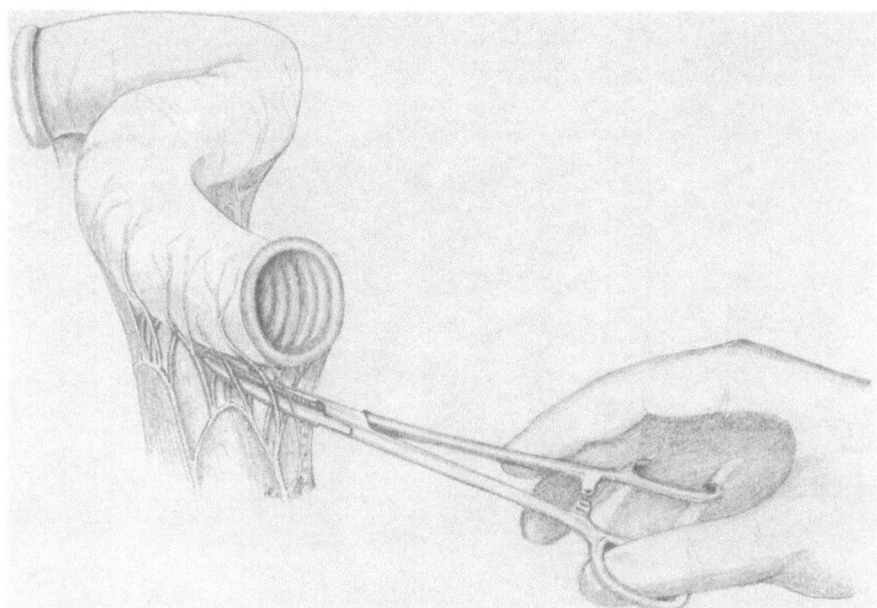

Fig. 1. Spreading of the mesenteric vessel arcades

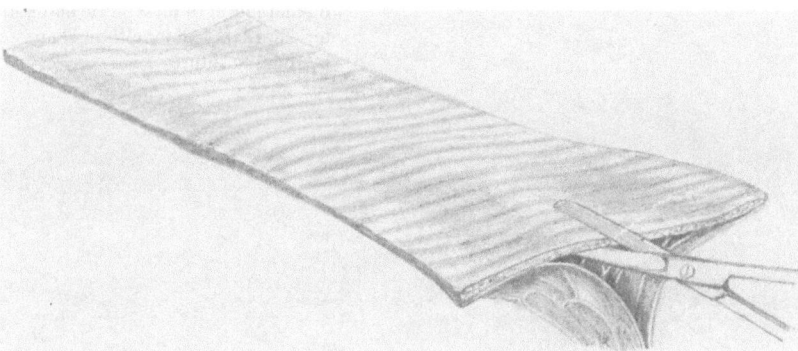

Fig. 2. After division of the antimesenteric border there follows division of the mesenteric border of the bowel wall with immediate haemostasis

Case Reports and Results

During the last 8 years we have seen four children with short bowel syndrome which resulted from an intrauterine volvulus in one case, from a congenital tumour of the mesenteric root in another case and from gastroschisis in two cases. One child had an additional colonic atresia and another was a conjoined twin. Our last child with a high terminal jejunostomy without remaining bowel died after 6

a

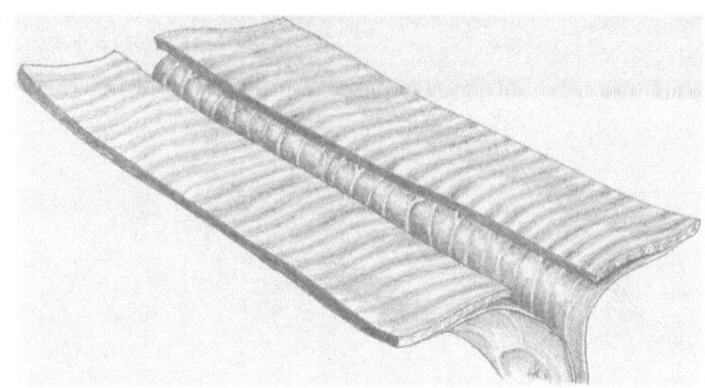

b

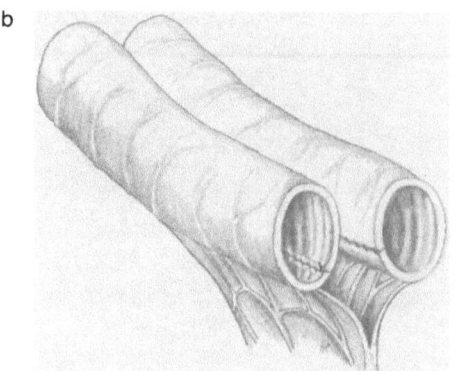

Fig. 3. a Finished longitudinal division.
b Adaptation of mesenteric and antimesenteric borders and longitudinal anastomosis by running sutures

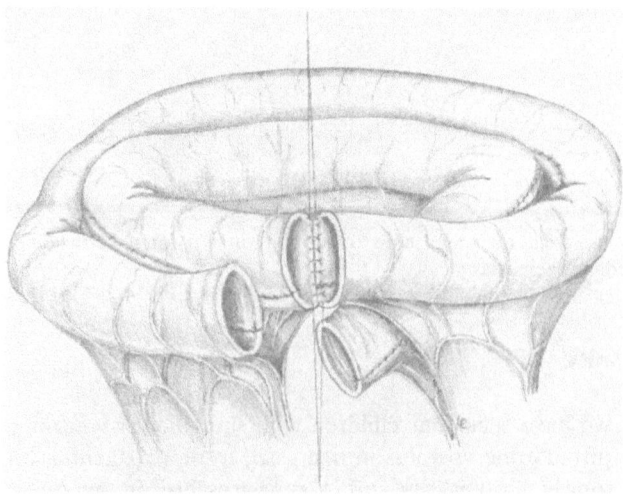

Fig. 4. Isoperistaltic series connection of the newly created bowel tubes and sling-like positioning to avoid tension on the mesenterium

months. The other three children recovered spontaneously and were able to come off TPN.

In a fifth case we looked for the possibility of surgical treatment when the child had reached the age of 2 years. Primarily, the child had a jejunal perforation 10 cm below the ligament of Treitz, caused by an intrauterine volvulus, with a remaining jejunum of 20 cm. Only the left half of the colon was present in this child. Enterostomies of the jejunal and colonic ends as well as of the perforated jejunum had been primarily established and a jejunocolostomy was performed secondarily. The enterostomy of the perforated jejunum was closed after several months. During the following months the remaining small bowel dilated massively without evidence of an anastomotic stenosis, so that peristalsis became ineffective. *Bacteroides* colonization and persistent overflow from the gastrostomy resulted. Repeated attempts to start oral feeding had to be stopped again and again. The child overcame several episodes of catheter sepsis. Strenuous and protracted efforts resulted finally in 100 ml tea per day as the only possible oral feeding. After 10 months of hospitalization the child went home during the day and was finally discharged for home TPN since the parents took care of her superbly. During the day the Hickman catheter remained closed; TPN was given exclusively at night.

The operation described was performed at the age of 25 months. Since the space between the bifurcated vessels at the mesenteric side of the bowel was too narrow for an instrumental anastomosis, longitudinal anastomosis between mesenteric and antimesenteric borders was carried out manually. Fitting the bowel loops into one another in a sling-like fashion gave tensionless series connection of both anastomosed bowel parts. The postoperative course was uneventful and bowel function began from the 2nd postoperative day. The girl was discharged 3 weeks later with the Hickman catheter, which she had had for 20 months still in place.

The girl is now 3 years of age and weighs 11 kg. She likes small amounts of noodles, mashed potato, savory snacks (salt sticks), spinach and sausage. In the meantime her tea intake has increased from 100 to 1500–1700 ml/day. Since her oral calorie intake is still insufficient, she needs administration of 600 ml glucose, 100 ml amino acids and 30 ml fat per day together with trace elements and vitamins via the Hickman catheter. Because of the huge oral fluid intake she passes stools frequently. It could well be that she could accept more oral feeding, but her problem is psychological since she has little experience of tasting or eating, and simply refuses to swallow the offered food. She is under psychotherapeutic care, oral food intake is increasing step by step and stool consistency is good. Thus, her prognosis is good, even if treatment is likely to be protracted. In the meantime she has come off TPN completely.

Discussion

Management of children with short bowel syndrome depends on two main problems: (a) the limited resorption function of the remaining bowel; and (b) the development of bowel dilatation with corresponding bowel dysfunction.

Both functions are connected with the length of the remaining bowel so short bowel syndrome must be defined precisely. The symptoms of short bowel syndrome may occur if 75–50 cm of small bowel remain, i.e. if about 70% of the original bowel length is missing. It must be recognized, however, that many errors may arise in the intraoperative measurement of bowel length: method of measurement, pre-tension of the bowel and quality of the bowel wall must be kept in mind. Above all, patients with necrotizing enterocolitis deserve particular attention, since pathohistological investigations reveal scarry changes of the bowel wall which limit resorption function considerably.

Single case reports in the literature hardly give insight into the real incidence of the short bowel syndrome. Mengel (personal communication) performed an inquiry on the incidence of short bowel syndrome regarding indications for small bowel transplantation in 1985. From 1975 to 1985, 19 of 34 paediatric surgical centres in the Federal Republic of Germany reported a total of 86 children with short bowel syndrome, our 5 cases included; 33 of them survived and 53 died. These figures emphasize the seriousness of the situation.

The different postoperative courses depend on the extent of the adaptation reaction. This reaction was extensively investigated by Clathworthy et al. [6] and Bähr and Flach [3]. Bowel adaptation is initiated by an increased functional load. It is characterized by hypertrophy, microscopically expressed in: (a) an increase in cell numbers in the mucosa in the sense of a true hyperplasia; (b) a cytologically increased cell migration; and (c) an increase in the number of stem cells and the frequency of cell cycles.

Resorption function of the bowel wall is intensified nonspecifically, by increase in enzyme activity and by other excretory mechanisms. High amounts of gastric juice and gastric acid shorten the transit time by hyperacidity. Bile and pancreatic excretions represent an important trophic factor. Experimentally, a deviation of bile into more distal bowel segments effects a hypertrophy of mucosal villi only below the point of deviation. Mucosal hypoplasia quickly developing under TPN can be prevented by simultaneous administration of cholecystokinin and secretin. The amount of remaining bowel limits the surface area for resorption of nutritive components. Missing bowel segments with different resorption tasks influence the prognosis. The ileocaecal valve and colon lengthen the transit time, so the extent of water and electrolyte resorption also determines the number of daily stools. Adaptation of the remaining short bowel to complete resorption is better the younger the child is. Macroscopically, bowel wall hyperplasia and hypertrophy expresses itself in the well-known wall thickening and dilatation [22]. A real bowel elongation, however, is unlikely and may occur to a minor extent only in neonates [3].

Adaptation abilities of jejunum, ileum and colon are different. Therefore, the amount of remaining bowel is of particular importance for the prognosis in these patients. Generally, the jejunum shows lesser adaptation than the ileum, even if there is a measurable increase of resorption. A missing ileum leads to a lack of specific resorptions, such as resorption of vitamin B_{12} and bile acids.

The colonic mucosa also reacts upon ileal resection with a persistent hyperplasia. However, this colonic reaction is only transient if jejunum is resected instead of ileum. According to Cummings [7, 8], the colon may even adapt so as to resorb short chain fatty acids in short bowel syndrome. Basically, hyperplasia within a bowel segment is more pronounced distally than proximally. This explains in our case why bowel adaptation and resorption showed only poor improvement. The remaining 20 cm of proximal jejunum represented a bowel segment where adaptation and resorption are by far the poorest.

Although the length of the remaining bowel plays an important role in prognosis, survival rate in our patient collective cannot be exclusively assessed by this parameter. Remarkably, the death rate was very high in multiple bowel atresia (15 of 23 infants) and gastroschisis (11 of 13 infants). The death rate was lower in infants with short bowel syndrome caused by a volvulus (8 of 16 infants) and even less in infants with necrotizing enterocolitis (6 of 16). Infants with gastroschisis and a remaining bowel of 20 cm plus the whole colon did not survive postoperatively. On the other hand, a bowel length of 8 cm plus the whole colon and 17 cm plus half of the colon was sufficient for full oral nutrition in two children with short bowel syndrome due to a volvulus. In general, a remaining bowel of 15–20 cm is the limit for oral nutrition, as found by Rickham et al. [16].

In order to improve or to speed oral calorie uptake, different operative techniques and procedures have been repeatedly recommended. As early as 1955, Hammer et al. [11] published the interposition of an antiperistaltic small bowel segment in animal experiments. The antiperistaltic segment should slow down the quick passage in a similar way to the preileal colonic interposition described by Hutcher et al. [14] in 1973. However, these interposed bowel segments had to be removed sooner or later because of recurrent bowel obstructions in almost all instances. Likewise, the vagotomy with pyloroplasty according to Frederik and Craig [10] and the recircling small bowel loop according to Altmann [2] were clinically unsuccessful, since peristalsis was disturbed unpredictably. In 1973 De Lorimier [9] described the trimming of the dilated small bowel which resulted in a considerably improved peristalsis and reduced bacterial overgrowth. In our opinion, the main drawback of this method is the removal of the mucosal surface in a situation where every square centimetre is urgently needed.

Our operative technique which was developed by Bianchi (1980) in pigs provides the following advantages. Small bowel length is doubled without loss of mucosal surface, but with simultaneous trimming of the mostly dilated bowel. Diminished bowel diameter renders peristalsis more effective which, above all, ensues isoperistaltically. Diminished bowel diameter and effective peristalsis prevent overgrowth with *Bacteroides*. Likewise, the diminished bowel diameter provides a closer contact between bowel contents and mucosa over a double length of passage, thus effecting a prolongation of contact and measurable transit time. In this way, oral feeding is facilitated and hospitalization is shortened.

Despite these clear advantages, the indication for this operation must be established individually from case to case. Since the procedure has not been standardized and sufficient experience has not been gathered, this technique must be considered a difficult one. Expected bowel adaptation and course of oral feeding should serve as criteria. If sufficient oral feeding is completely impossible or if it improves very slowly, this operation may well be indicated. If an extremely long time to establish oral feedings can be expected, the operation should not in our opinion, be postponed until it becomes unavoidable later on. The operation according to Bianchi is also indicated if technical problems in TPN arise (difficult venous access).

We have found only three case reports in the literature where the technique had been applied successfully. The first child with a gastroschisis and a remaining small bowel of 39 cm was reported by Boeckman and Traylor [5] and the second child with a gastroschisis, 25 cm of jejunum and half of the colon by Agrain et al. [1]. A third case of a girl with multiple small bowel atresias and a remaining bowel consisting of 10 cm of jejunum, 24 cm of ileum and a complete colon was described by Thompson et al. [18] in 1985.

The discussion of operative technique concentrates on longitudinal division of the mesenteric border of the bowel wall, since it depends on the vessel free space between the bifurcated vessel levels. Sufficient space for introduction of a straight stapler for division and instrumental longitudinal anastomosis may possibly be found in older children or in those with extreme bowel dilatation. The advantage of a stapler is division and anastomosis with minimal blood loss. In more restricted spaces a stepwise, manual procedure with running sutures must be employed. It must be kept in mind that the afferent arteries represent terminal arteries in this situation.

Positioning of the divided bowel parts to be connected in series is another technically important point. It is extremely important to avoid any tension on the afferent vessels. Spiral positioning of both bowel parts seem to be most advantageous. Internal drainage or splinting is not necessary. As in the other publications, we did not observe anastomotic leakage and there was a radiologically verifiable peristalsis. Length of follow-up, clinical course and the possibility of oral feeding must be individually weighed against the risks of this operation. However, all children who underwent this procedure improved quickly in their calorie uptake.

References

1. Agrain Y, Cornet D, Cezard JP, Boureau M (1985) Longitudinal division of small intestine: a surgical possibility for children with the very short bowel syndrome. Z Kinderchir 40:233
2. Altmann GG (1965) Demonstration of a morphological control mechanism in the small intestine: role of pancreatic secretions and bile intestinal adaption. Dowling, Riecken. Schattauer, Stuttgart, pp 75–86
3. Bähr R, Flach A (1978) Morphological and functional adaption after massive resection of small intestine: experiments using minipigs of the Göttingen strain. Prog Pediatr Surg 12:107
4. Bianchi A (1980) Intestinal loop lengthening – a technique for increasing small intestine length. J Pediatr Surg 15:145
5. Boeckman CR, Traylor R (1981) Bowel lengthening for short gut syndrome. J Pediatr Surg 16:996
6. Clathworthy HW, Saleeby R, Lovingood C (1952) Extensive small bowel resection in young dogs. Its effect on growth and development. Surg 32:341

7. Cummings JH (1981) Short chain fatty acids in the human colon. Gut 22:763
8. Cummings JH, James W, Wiggins HS (1973) Role of the colon in ileal resection diarrhoea. Lancet i:344
9. De Lorimier A (1973) Discussion: proximal jejunoplasty in the treatment of jejunal atresia. Pediatr Surg 8:685
10. Frederik PL, Craig TV (1964) Effect of vagotomy and pyloroplasty on weight loss and survival of dogs after massive intestinal resection. Surgery 56:135
11. Hammer JM, Seay PH, Hill EJ (1955) Intestinal segments as internal pedicle grafts. Arch Surg 71:625
12. Hughes CA, Ducker DA: Adaptation of the small intestine – does it occur in man? Scand J Gastroenterol [Suppl] 17:149
13. Hughes CA (1982) Intestinal adaption in neonatal gastroenterology. Tanner u. Stocks Edition: Intercept, Newcastle upon Tyne
14. Hutcher NE, Mendez-Picon G, Salzberg AM (1973) Prejejunal transposition of colon to prevent the developement of short bowel syndrome in puppies. J Pediatr Surg 8:771
15. Kurz R, Sauer H (1983) Treatment and metabolic findings in extreme short bowel syndrome with 11 cm jejunal remnant. J Pediatr Surg 18:257
16. Rickham PP, Irving I, Shmerling D (1977) Long term results following extensive small intestinal resection in the neonatal period. Prog Pediatr Surg 10:65
17. Ricour C. Duhamel JF, Nihoul-Fekete C (1985) Enteral and parenteral nutrition in the short bowel syndrome in children. World J Surg 9:310
18. Thompson JS, Vanderhoof JA, Antonson D (1985) Intestinal tapering and lengthening for short bowel syndrome. J Pediatr Gastroenterol Nutr 4:495
19. Tilson MD (1980) Pathophysiology and treatment of short bowel syndrome. Surg Clin North Am 60:1273
20. Weber TR, Vane DW, Grosfield JL (1982) Tapering enteroplasty in infants with bowel atresia and short gut. Arch Surg 117:684
21. Williamson RCN (1978) Intestinal adaption, structural, functional and cytokinetic changes. N Engl J Med 298:1393
22. Williamson RCN (1982) Intestinal adaption: factors that influence morphology. Scand J Gastroenterol [Suppl] 17:21
23. Wilmore WD (1972) Factors correlating with a successful outcome following extensive intestinal resection in newborn infants. J Pediatr 80:88

Small Bowel Transplantation: Report of a Clinical Case

E. Deltz, W. Mengel, and H. Hamelmann

Summary

Extensive small bowel resection may become necessary for several reasons in children and adults. The only causal therapy of short bowel syndrome is small bowel transplantation. So far severe immunological problems have caused deleterious results despite technically successful transplantation. A clinical case of small bowel transplantation in a child is reported. The 3-year-old boy had been operated on for volvulus which had led to nearly total gangrene of the whole small bowel. Finally, only 4 cm of jejunum could be saved. Total parenteral nutrition (TPN) therefore became necessary. Small bowel transplantation was carried out with the mother as donor; transplantation technique is described in detail. Postoperative immunosuppression was performed by administration of cyclosporin A and prednisolone. Because of graft rejection, the graft had to be removed on the 12th postoperative day. At present, the child is well and on TPN again. This case shows that small bowel transplantation by living related organ donation is technically possible without impairment of the donor's quality of life. Further experimental and clinical work should be encouraged.

Zusammenfassung

Aus verschiedenen Gründen kann eine ausgedehnte Dünndarmresektion beim Kind und Erwachsenen nötig werden. Die Dünndarmtransplantation ist die einzige kausale Therapie des Kurzdarmsyndroms. Trotz technisch erfolgreicher Transplantationen führten bisher schwere immunologische Probleme zu ungünstigen Ergebnissen. Über einen klinischen Fall von Dünndarmtransplantation bei einem Kind wird berichtet. Der 3jährige Junge mußte wegen eines Volvulus operiert werden, der zu einer fast vollständigen Dünndarmgangrän geführt hatte. Letztlich konnten nur 4 cm Jejunum gerettet werden, und das Kind mußte parenteral ernährt werden. Es wurde eine Dünndarmtransplantation mit der Mutter als Spenderin durchgeführt.

Die Operationstechnik wird ausführlich beschrieben. Die postoperative Immunsuppression erfolgte mit Cyclosporin A und Prednisolon. Wegen einer Abstoßungsreaktion mußte das Transplantat am 12. postoperativen Tag entfernt werden. Gegenwärtig wird das Kind wieder parenteral ernährt und ist in einem guten Zustand. Dieser Fall zeigt, daß die Dünndarmtransplantation mit einem Spenderorgan eines lebenden Verwandten ohne Beeinträchtigung der Lebensqualität des Spenders technisch möglich ist. Weitere experimentelle und klinische Forschungsarbeiten sollten erfolgen.

Résumé

Pour plusieurs raisons, une résection de l'intestin grêle, tant chez l'enfant que chez l'adulte, peut être indispensable. La transplantation de l'intestin grêle est la seule thérapie envisageable dans le

Chirurgische Klinik, Christian Albrechts University Kiel, Arnold-Heller-Strasse 7, D-2300 Kiel, Federal Republic of Germany

Progress in Pediatric Surgery, Vol. 25
Angerpointner (Ed.)
© Springer-Verlag Berlin Heidelberg 1990

cas d'une atrophie intestinale. Jusqu'à ce jour se posait, comme pour toute transplantation, le problème du rejet. Nous rapportons un cas de transplantation intestinale chez un enfant. Le nouveau-né devait impérativement être opéré d'un volvulus d'un intestin grêle quasiment gangréneux. Seuls 4 cm de jéjunum pouvaient être sauvés et l'enfant nécessitait une alimentaion parentérale. Une transplantation intestinale avec la mère comme donneuse fut entreprise. La technique opératoire est décrite en détails. Le rejet a été combattu en post-opération par de la cyclosporine A et de la prednisolone. Etant donné une manisfestation de rejet, le greffon a dû être excisé au 12 ème jour. Parallèlement, l'enfant fut remis sous nutrition parentérale et son état s'est stabilisé. Ce cas montre que la transplantation d'intestin grêle à partir d'un donneur vivant, membre de la famille, est techniquement possible. Travaux en cours.

Introduction

Extensive small bowel resection may become necessary for several reasons in children and adults. In adult patients obstruction of mesenteric vessels caused by thrombosis or embolic occlusion of arteries or venous thrombosis causes bowel gangrene which has to be treated by resection of extensive parts of the small bowel. Widespread involvement of small bowel in Crohn's disease is another reason for extensive resection of small bowel. In contrast, in infants and children connatal abnormalities are usually the underlying causes for extensive small bowel resection. Gangrene of small bowel caused by volvulus in cases of malrotation, mesenterium commune or multiple atretic segments can be treated only by resection of small bowel, thus causing short bowel syndrome which in cases of insufficient length and adaptation of the small bowel remnant makes total parenteral nutrition (TPN) necessary.

The technique of TPN has been very successful in the last 10 years [2, 3, 11, 12], but patients on TPN are still threatened by severe septic complications caused by permanent intravenous catheters or the side effects of parenteral nutrition such as metabolic disturbances of the liver, including cholestasis, gallstone formation, bone demineralization and pancreatitis, or the consequences of gastric hyperacidity and hypersecretion [12].

The only causal therapy of short bowel syndrome caused by small bowel loss consists in replacement of the missing organ, i.e. small bowel transplantation. The urgent need of this treatment led to the first attempts at clinical small bowel transplantation. After the first case in 1967 [7], a few attempts were made in the early 1970's [5], but all these operations led to the patient's death.

Despite the successful course of these operations from the technical point of view, the severe immunological problems which are encountered in allogeneic small bowel transplantation caused the deleterious results. These complex immunological problems stimulated extensive basic research on the immunological fundamentals of small bowel transplantation. The result of these efforts was the basic knowledge of mechanisms of graft rejection [4, 6] anti-host reactions (graft-versus-host reaction, GVHR) which presents a specific immunological problem in small bowel transplantation [1, 9]. The development of methods which made possible manipulation and suppression of both rejection and anti-host reactions [1], has led to new attempts at clinical small bowel transplantation (Z. Cohen 1985, personal communication; Ricour 1987, personal communication), which unfortunately have been unsuccessful until now. Against this background and based on own extensive experimental studies we made our first attempt at clinical small bowel transplantation.

Case History

The patient, a boy born in 1983 had to undergo nearly total small bowel resection after development of small bowel gangrene caused by a volvulus in the mesenterium commune. The small bowel − except for 6 cm of upper jejunum and the ascending colon − and the right hemicolon were resected. A jejunostoma was formed. Reanastomosing of jejunum and colon transversum was carried out 2 weeks after primary resection. After resection of an anastomotic stenosis a remnant of 4 cm jejunum distal of the ligament of Treitz could be saved. Under these circumstances sufficient enteral nutrition could not be established, despite persistent attempts so that continuous TPN had to be carried out, performed in the clinic at night; the boy was allowed to go home for 8 h during the day.

Despite long-term hospitalization and application of nutrient solutions by expert nurses and doctors, several septic episodes with almost lethal outcome occurred. Therefore, we performed a small bowel transplantation with living related organ donation by the mother of the patient on 5 November 1987. HL-A typing showed haploidentity and identity in two other antigens, including DR. On the day prior to operation the donor's and recipient's gastrointestinal tracts were prepared by whole gut irrigation.

Operative Technique

Donor Operation

A segment of midjejunum of the recipient's mother was selected by checking the vascular architecture of mesenterium by diaphanoscopy of the mesenterium. The

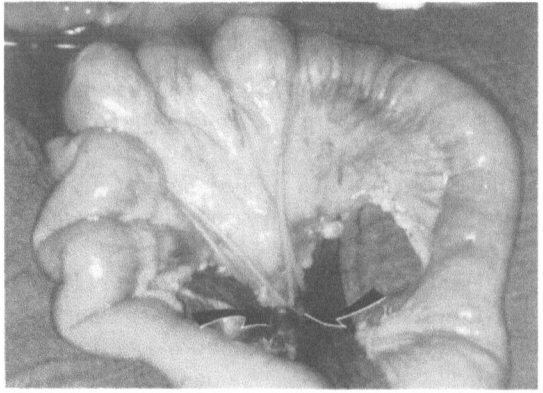

Fig. 1. Midjejunal segment of the donor (*arrows* indicate mesenteric vessels)

mesenteric vein and artery were then prepared up to their origin from upper mesenteric or ileocolic artery or vein respectively (Fig. 1). A segment of length 80 cm was removed after closing the bowel at both ends and after dissection with a GIA stapling device and transection of the vessels after proximal ligation. Continuity of donor small bowel was reestablished by an end-to-end anastomosis with a single layer interrupted suture. The graft was removed from the donor and vas-

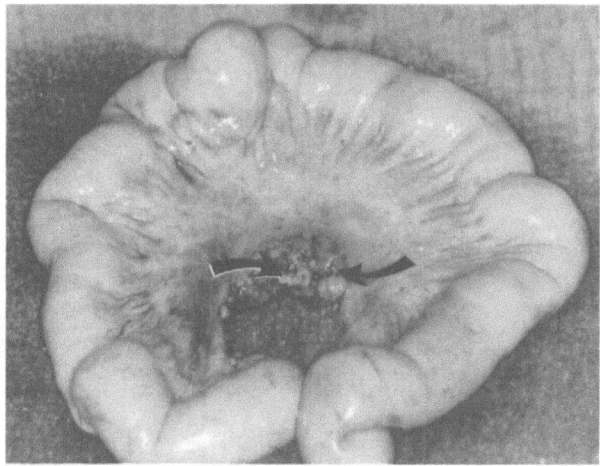

Fig. 2. Small bowel graft after perfusion (*arrows* indicate vascular pedicle)

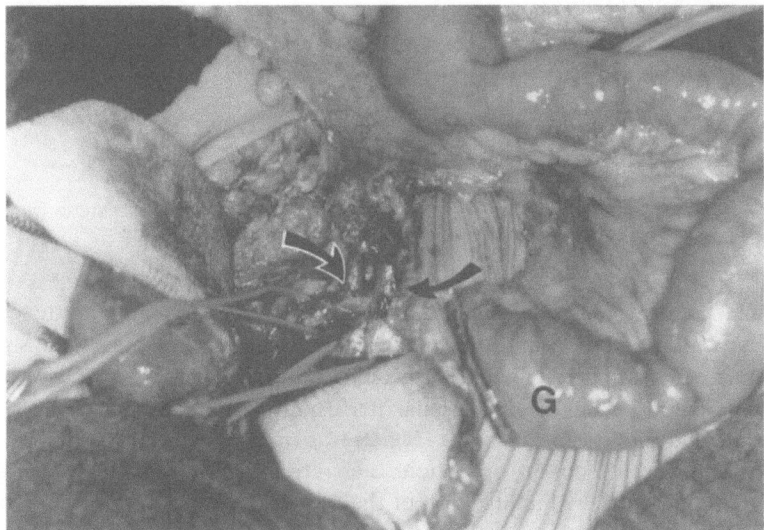

Fig. 3. Small bowel graft *(G)* in situ with vessel anastomoses *(arrows)* completed

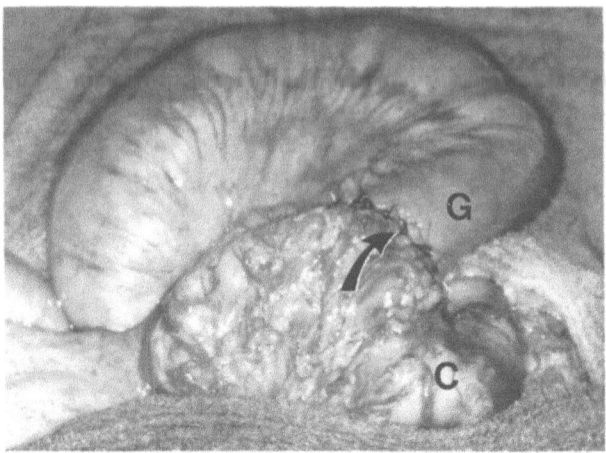

Fig. 4. Anastomosis *(arrow)* of the aboral end of the graft *(G)* to recipient's colon *(C)*

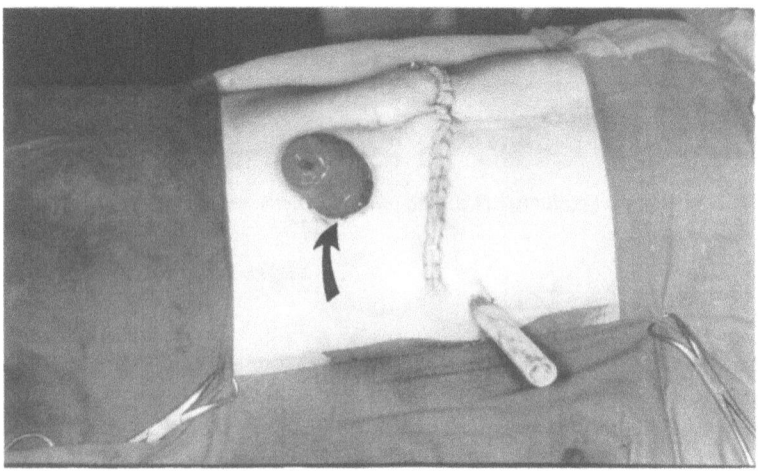

Fig. 5. Recipient after closure of laparotomy. Oral end of the graft exteriorized as a stoma *(arrow)*

cular perfusion started after cannulation of the mesenteric artery with 4°C Eurocollins solution until the effluent was clear. The lumen of the small bowel graft was also perfused with Eurocollins solution. Thus, remnants of bowel contents could be removed. Vascular perfusion started 5 min after removal of the graft. After perfusion the graft (Fig. 2) was transferred to the recipient.

During the donor operation the recipient was prepared by transverse laparotomy and by mobilization of the jejunocolic anastomosis and mobilization of the left colon to the right of the patient. Common iliac vein and artery had been prepared for the anastomoses. After cross-clamping of the vessels an end-to-side anastomosis of the mesenteric vein of the graft to the common iliac vein and the mesenteric artery to the common iliac artery by a running 8–0 suture was performed (Fig. 3). After removal of the clamp the graft showed good perfusion. Its colour was light red, like a normal gut segment. Total ischaemic time was 1 h 20 min. The warm ischaemic time was 40 min. As there were no circulatory problems nor any signs of rejection the distal end of the graft, after resection of 10 cm at both ends, was anastomosed to the colon transversum of the recipient 3 cm distal of the jejunocolic anastomoses (Fig. 4). The oral end of the graft was exteriorized as a stoma. The graft was placed to the left abdomen and the laparotomy closed (Fig. 5).

Clinical Course

The first postoperative days were uneventful. The boy recovered from the operation and was well. Immunosuppression was performed by 10 mg/kg cyclosporin A and 45 mg prednisolone. The mucosa of the graft which was visible at the stoma appeared normal. The biopsies taken from the stoma showed a normal histological picture. On the 5th postoperative day body temperature increased and histological analysis revealed mononuclear infiltration of the graft as a sign of rejection. Macroscopically the mucosa showed a slight oedema and its colour was blueish red. Rejection therapy was therefore started by treatment with 100 mg prednisolone and 3 mg/kg anti-thymocyte globulin (ATG).

On the 7th postoperative day the clinical state was bad. Body temperature remained high (39°C). Therefore relaparotomy was performed, but the graft showed only a slight oedema of the bowel wall and mesenterium. Therefore, removal of the graft was not judged to be necessary. Rejection therapy by ATG and prednisolone was continued, but the clinical state of the recipient remained bad. Histology taken by a gastroscope via the stoma now showed granulomatous infiltration with severe damage of the mucosa. As the clinical state deteriorated and a large amount of fluid was lost through the stoma the graft had to be removed on the 12th postoperative day. The colonic incision of the anastomosis was closed by direct suture. After removal of the graft the boy recovered quickly. Fever disappeared and wound healing was normal. Histological evaluation of the graft showed a severe rejection by infiltration of all layers of the bowel wall with loss of mucosa. Thrombotic material occluding the vessels of the graft contained immune complexes, thus giving evidence of a humoral rejection reaction in addition to prevailing cellular infiltration. At present the recipient is well and on TPN again. The donor shows no impairment of intestinal function.

Discussion

The case shows that small bowel transplantation with living related organ donation is possible from the technical point of view without impairment of the donor's quality of life. Close monitoring of the graft by biopsies makes it possible to determine the type and strength of rejection and to assess the effectiveness of rejection therapy. Interpretation of histological findings can be correlated with experimental data [6, 8–10].

Our observations show that rejection mechanisms in clinical small bowel transplantation are identical to those which have been investigated in rodents and large animals. In spite of the fact that rejection in this case could not be treated successfully, our clinical observation shows that, if based on experimental results, clinical small bowel transplantation is no longer a life-threatening procedure. This case of unsuccessful small bowel transplantation, but with unimpaired survival of donor and recipient, should encourage further experimental and clinical work in the field of small bowel transplantation.

References

1. Deltz E, Ulrichs K, Schack T, Friedrichs B, Müller-Ruchholtz W, Müller-Hermelink HK, Thiede A (1986) Graft-versus-host reaction in small-bowel transplantation and possibilities for its circumvention. Am J Surg 151:379–386
2. Dorney St FA, Ament ME, Berquist WE, Vargas JH, Hassall E (1985) Improved survival in very short small bowel of infancy with use of long-term parenteral nutrition. J Pediatr 107:521–525
3. Grosfeld JL, Rescoria FJ, West KW (1986) Short bowel syndrome in infancy and childhood. Am J Surg 151:41–46
4. Hardy MA, Chabot J, Tannenbaum G, Benvenisty AJ (1986) Graft acceptance: modification of immunogenicity of the donor or the donor organ with or without host immunosuppression. In: Deltz E, Thiede A, Hamelmann H (eds) Small-bowel transplantation. Springer, Berlin Heidelberg New York Tokyo, pp 135–152
5. Hardy MA, Iga CH, Lau H (1985) Intestinal transplantation: laboratory experience and clinical consequences. In: Thiede A, Deltz E, Engemann R, Hamelmann H (eds) Microsurgical models in rats for transplantation research. Springer, Berlin Heidelberg New York Tokyo, pp 337–346
6. Liedgens P, Müller-Hermelink HK, Deltz E (1986) Rejection in heterotopic small-bowel transplantation. In: Deltz E, Thiede A, Hamelmann H (eds) Small-bowel transplantation. Springer, Berlin Heidelberg New York Tokyo, pp 116–120
7. Nordgren S, Cohen Z (1986) Intestinal transplantation: surgical techniques in animals and man. In: Deltz E, Thiede A, Hamelmann H (eds) Small-bowel transplantation. Springer, Berlin Heidelberg New York Tokyo, pp 172–181
8. Revillon Y, Gallix P, Arnaud-Battandier F, Ricour C (1986) Small-bowel allotransplantation in pigs using cyclosporine A: technique and results. In: Deltz E, Thiede A, Hamelmann H (eds) Small-bowel transplantation. Springer, Berlin Heidelberg New York Tokyo, pp 192–195
9. Schraut WH, Lee KK (1985) Clinicopathologic differentiation of rejection and graft-vs-host disease following small-bowel transplantation. In: Deltz E, Thiede A, Hamelmann H (eds) Small-bowel transplantation. Springer, Berlin Heidelberg New York Tokyo, pp 98–108
10. Stauffer UG (1986) Monitoring of small-bowel grafts by mucosal suction biopsies. In: Deltz E, Thiede A, Hamelmann H (eds) Small-bowel transplantation. Springer, Berlin Heidelberg New York Tokyo, pp 234–240
11. Vargas J-H, Ament ME, Berquist WE (1987) Long-term home parenteral nutrition in pediatrics: ten years of experience in 102 patients. J Pediatr Gastroenterol Nutr 6:24–32
12. Wolman SL, Jeejeebhoy KN, Stewart S, Greig PD (1986) Experience in home parenteral nutrition and indications for small-bowel transplantation. In: Deltz E, Thiede A, Hamelmann H (eds) Small-bowel transplantation. Springer, Berlin Heidelberg New York Tokyo, pp 214–221

Deep Anterior Resection with Circular Stapled Anastomosis of Congenital Megacolon: Clinical Results

P. Dohrmann, W. Mengel, and H. Schaube

Summary

This report deals with instrumental suture in the deep anterior rectum resection when treating Hirschsprung's disease. The concept includes: ensuring diagnosis, cleaning the intestines, antibiotic prophylaxis, intraoperative testing of the anastomosis and postoperative X-ray by a standardized technique. Our first experience in the use of the stapler was gained with ten patients. One case of anastomosis insufficiency occurred. With the stapler apparatus, safe anastomosis was possible. The stapler facilitates anastomoses in deep resections. Therefore, a deep resection of the pathological segment in Hirschsprung's disease is possible. The practicality of the stapler and the favourable clinical experience justify the continued application of the instrumental suture technique in children's surgery.

Zusammenfassung

Es wird über die Instrumentenanastomose zur tiefen anterioren Rektumresektion bei der Behandlung des M. Hirschsprung berichtet. Das Behandlungskonzept umfaßt Diagnosesicherung, Darmspülung, Antibiotikaprophylaxe, intraoperative Testung der Anastomosensuffizienz und postoperative standardisierte Röntgenkontrolle der Anastomose. Erste Erfahrungen mit dem EEA-Stapler wurden bei 10 Patienten gesammelt. Dabei trat 1 Fall von Anastomoseninsuffizienz auf. Eine sichere Anastomosierung mit dem Stapler war möglich. Der Stapler erleichtert die Anastomose bei der tiefen Resektion, so daß das aganglionäre Segment beim M. Hirschsprung sehr tief abgesetzt werden kann.

Praktikabilität und gute klinische Ergebnisse lassen die klinische Anwendung der Instrumentenanastomose auch bei Kindern angeraten erscheinen.

Résumé

Nous rapportons les cas d'anastomose lors d'une résection rectale profonde au décours d'une maladie de Hirschsprung. La thérapeutique comprend: une confirmation du diagnostic, un lavement, une antibiothérapie de protection, une vérification per- et post-opératoire de la solidité des sutures et un contrôle radiologique standard de l'anastomose. Les premières expériences avec le "EEA stapler" ont été effectuées sur 10 patients. Dans un cas, nous avons eu un défaut de suture. La sûreté de la suture a été rendue possible grâce au stapler. Le stapler facilite les sutures dans les cas de résections larges, de telle sorte que le segment aganglionnaire de la maladie de Hirschsprung peut être largement réséqué.

L'utilisation partique et les bons résultats cliniques justifient l'anomastose également en chirurgie infantile.

Division of Paediatric Surgery, Department of Surgery, Christian Albrechts University Kiel, Arnold-Heller-Strasse 7, D-2300 Kiel, Federal Republic of Germany

Progress in Pediatric Surgery, Vol. 25
Angerpointner (Ed.)
© Springer-Verlag Berlin Heidelberg 1990

Introduction

Following a deep rectum resection of an intestinal segment, four procedures can be applied to re-establish continuity: end-to-end, side-to-side and end-to-side anastomosis as well as a so-called passage. In deep anterior resection, end-to-end anastomosis is used most often, because it re-establishes nearly physiological conditions [7]. Of the different manual suture techniques the single-row, all-layer adaption on the edge yields the best results in regard to revascularization, suture sufficiency and stenosis rate [5]. In the last few years, the stapler apparatus has become increasingly important with the aim of making anastomoses simpler, quicker and safer. The first stapler apparatus was developed by Victor Fischer in cooperation with the Hungarian surgeon Humer Hültle [6] in 1908. This was a linear suture apparatus which made possible an everting anastomosis. Encouraged by the developments at the Sklifossowsky Institute in Moscow [8], the United Surgical Corporation developed suture instruments with exchangeable, disposable stapler magazines which allowed circular anastomoses. The remarkable thing about these apparatus is that the staplers do not crush, but unite tissue so that even distal of the staple row the blood circulation in the tissue is maintained. The scientific test of the utility of the suture instruments in the gastrointestinal area was the subject of numerous studies [1, 2, 10]. After good experience in adult surgery it seemed justified to use them in children's surgery. This paper reports our experience with the circular stapler suture in operations for congenital megacolon.

Patients and Method

In our clinic a deep resection with the EEA (entero-enteric-anastomosis) stapler was performed on ten children. The patients were between 6 and 10 months of age, (median 6.8 months). In six children a preternatural anus was established after diagnosis at birth. For the remaining four patients the diagnosis was made only in infancy and primarily resected.

Tractical Concept

1. Ensuring diagnosis by defecogram, histology and acetylcholinesterase determination
2. Cleansing of bowels with oral liquid food and enema
3. Systematic ultra-short antibiotic prophylaxis, 2×100 mg/kg cefotaxime
4. Test of primary anastomosis sufficiency by transanal instillation of liquid
5. Test of completeness of the tissue rings in the machine head
6. Checking anastomosis on the 8th–12th postoperative day with Peritrast
7. Bougienage programme from the 3rd postoperative day with Hegar pins
8. Systematic follow-up and renewed X-ray with contrast media containing BaSO4

Technical Procedure

The EEA stapler manufactured by the Auto-Suture Company was used; staple magazines are available in three sizes:

EEA 31, green magazine: outer diameter (o.d.) 31 mm; inner diameter (i.d.) 21 mm
EEA 28, blue magazine: o.d. 28 mm; i.d. 18 mm
EEA 25, white magazine: o.d. 25 mm; i.d. 15 mm
as well as the disposable instrument
C-D-EEA 21: o.d. 21 mm; i.d. 11 mm

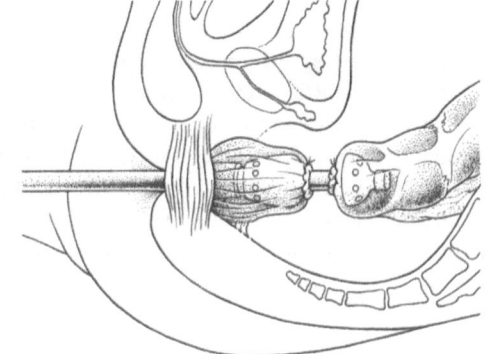

Fig. 1. Low anterior resection with circular stapled anastomosis. Position of the EEA instrument before the final adaptation of the colon stumps

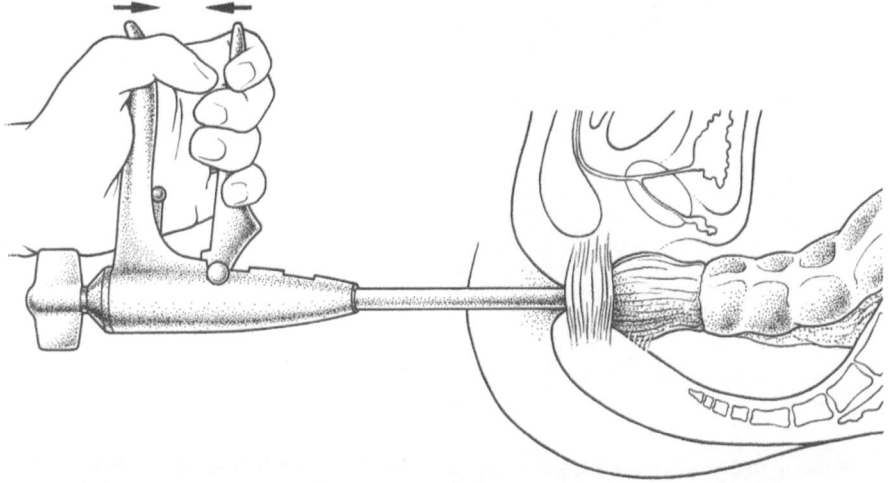

Fig. 2. Low anterior resection with circular stapled anastomosis. The EEA stapler is closed and activated to make the circular, end-to-end inverting anastomosis

In transanal employment, a circular inverted two-row staple suture is achieved. On removal of the stapler, assuming technically correct use and after testing the sufficiency of the anastomosis, no other sutures are required (Figs. 1 and 2).

Results

For three children the extent of resection involved the rectosigmoid, in three patients parts of the colon descendens also had to be resected and in one child it was necessary to place the proximal edge of resection into the centre of the colon transversum. For all ten children the white staple magazine with an outer diameter of 25 mm was used. The depth of anastomosis (measured at the anocutaneous line) was 3–5 cm (average 3.9 cm). There were no complications concerning the technical performance of the anastomosis with the stapler. In one case the staple suture caught in an abdominal towel, necessitating resuturing by hand. Intraoperative testing of anastomosis tightness by transanal instillation of liquid showed no insufficiency in any patient.

Postoperative bougienage started on the 3rd postoperative day. Here there appeared to be a pronounced inclination to shrinkage. The bougienage took place twice daily with an increase of bougie size by 1 Charrière per week, up to 13–14 Charrière according to age. The bougienage (after hospital treatment) was then continued by the mother at home once a day.

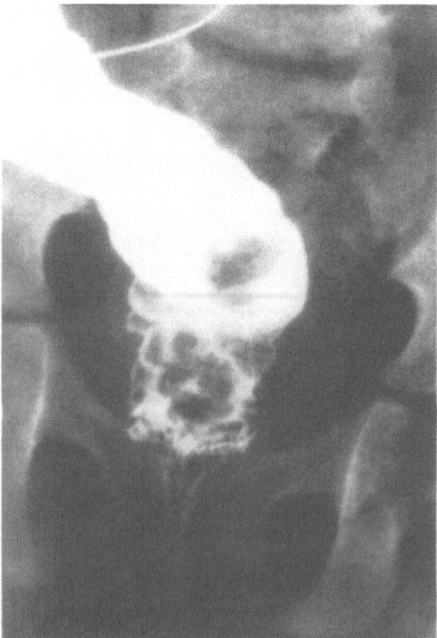

Fig. 3. X-ray follow-up 1 year after low anterior resection. A 2.5-cm stapled anastomosis in a 1½-year-old boy with congenital megacolon

Primary postoperative follow-up of the anastomoses on the 8th–12th day resulted for nine children in a sufficient anastomosis; in one child a small leak was found. In four children the first follow-up examination after discharge from hospital 4 weeks postoperatively made manual stretching of the sphincter necessary. Some 11 months after surgery one patient developed an adhesion ileus which required renewed surgical intervention. After 1 year the pronounced cicatricial ring at the site of anastomosis was no longer to be found in any of the children. X-ray examination after 12 months showed good elasticity of the anastomosis and an unrestricted depletion of the rectum (Fig. 3). One patient who already required surgery for an adhesion ileus had to have a preternatural anus installed after the occurrence of an ileus with severe enterocolitis.

Discussion

With the reservation appropriate to the low number of cases, the results prove that safe anastomoses are possible with the stapler apparatus. In one of ten patients an insufficiency of the anastomosis was found radiologically which was cured with conservative therapy. The prerequisites for a successful instrumental anastomosis are manifold and correspond to those of a manual suture [9]. Besides an adaptation free of tension and good blood circulation, careful preparation of the intestinal ends is essential.

In adult rectum surgery Beart and Kelly [1] proved in a randomized comparative study the equal value of single-row manual and EEA sutures. With the EEA the anastomosis time was shortened and for ten patients the sphincter was maintained, which would have been impossible with manual suture; thus, the range of indications has been extended. Similar results were achieved by Thiede et al. [11] in a controlled study on deep rectum resection of adults, comparing the manual with the instrumental suture. The clinical results were nearly indentical; however, the circular suture instrument allowed extended indications of rectum resection, especially in men with a narrow pelvis. Gordon [4] presented a technique, using the curved EEA stapler for the Duhamel procedure, which has further facilitated the performance of this operation.

Our experience shows that the EEA stapler is suitable for rectum anastomoses in childhood. In regard to handling technique the stapler especially facilitates anastomosis in deep resection by allowing a greater radicalization for removal of the pathological segment, especially in Hirschsprung's disease. We had a subjective impression of a more pronounced tendency to shrinkage. Thus, we began the bougienage programme in cases of instrumental anastomosis on the 3rd postoperative day. This tendency to shrinkage was also observed with rectum anastomoses in adult surgery, here, caused by the use of too small a magazine [10]. In the case of our infants, however, the lumen size of the rectum limits the use of larger magazines. Bleedings from the anastomoses when using the stapler machine have been described by Fischer [3]. These must be observed carefully and, should they occur, must be corrected immediately during surgery. We never observed secondary stenosis as the sole reaction to the metal implants.

References

1. Beart RW, Kelly KA (1981) Randomized prospective evaluation of the EEA stapler for colorectal anastomoses. Am J Surg 141:143–147
2, Becker H, Probst M, Ungeheur E (1980) Die maschinelle Anastomose nach anteriorer Rektumresektion. Chirurg 51:341–343
3. Fischer MG (1976) Bleeding from stapler anastomosis. Am J Surg 131:745–747
4. Gordon PH (1983) An improved technique for the Duhamel operation using the EEA stapler. Dis Colon Rectum 26:690–692
5. Hell K, Allgöwer M (1976) Die Colonresektion. Springer, Berlin Heidelberg New York, pp 59–70
6. Hültl H (1908) Kongreß der ungarischen Gesellschaft für Chirurgie. Pester Med Chir Presse 45:108–110, 121–122
7. Junginger T, Pichelmaier H (1982) Nahtmaterialien und Nahttechniken in der Colonchirurgie. In: Thiede A, Hamelmann H (eds) Nahtmaterialien und Nahttechniken. Springer, Berlin Heidelberg New York, pp 288–295
8. Katalina TV (1964) The use of the apparatuses PKS 25 and SK in the clinic, in mechanical sutures in surgery of the gastrointestinal tract. Sklifossowsky Institute, Moscow
9. Knight CD, Griffen FD (1983) Techniques of low rectal reconstruction. Curr Probl Surg 20:388–456
10. Thiede A, Jostarndt L, Troidl H, Poser HL, Hamelmann H (1981) Der Wert der zirkulären maschinellen Colon- und Rectumanastomose (EEA). Chirurg 52:30–35
11. Thiede A, Schubert G, Poser HL, Jostarndt L (1984) Zur Technik der Rectumanastomosen bei Rectumresektionen. Chirurg 55:326–355

Secondary Sagittal Posterior Anorectoplasty

A. M. Holschneider

Summary

From October 1984 to December 1986, 25 continence-improving operations were performed at the Paediatric Surgical Clinic of the Children's Hospital, Cologne. Smooth muscle inversion plasties were carried out during abdominosacroperineal pull-through procedures in eight neonates. Anterior sagittal anorectoplasties were employed in four female neonates. Secondary continence-improving procedures had to be carried out in 13 patients, with secondary sagittal anterior rectoplasties in 5 instances and posterior sagittal anorectoplasties in another 7 instances. Gracilis transposition according to Pickrell was employed in one boy. Among the seven children who underwent posterior sagittal rectoplasty, there were four patients where remnants of earlier gracilis or gluteus maximus plasties could be additionally used for creation of a continent sphincter apparatus. Among the 13 older patients with secondary continence-improving operations, 7 achieved complete continence and 6 markedly improved continence effecting continence for solid and pultaceous stools, but soiling under stress and diarrhoea. No child remained entirely incontinent.

Zusammenfassung

Von Oktober 1984 bis Ende 1986 wurden an der Kinderchirurgischen Klinik der Städtischen Kinderklinik Köln 25 kontinenzverbessernde Operationen durchgeführt. Bei 8 Neugeborenen wurde eine glattmuskuläre Umstülpplastik im Rahmen eines abdominosakroperinealen Durchzugverfahrens vorgenommen. Bei 4 weiblichen Neugeborenen wurde eine anteriore sagittale Anorektoplastik vorgenommen. Sekundäre kontinenzverbessernde Eingriffe erfolgten bei 13 Patienten, wobei 5mal eine sekundäre sagittale anteriore Rektoplastik sowie 7mal eine posteriore sagittale Anorektoplastik durchgeführt wurde. Bei einem Knaben wurde eine Gracilistransposition nach Pickrell vorgenommen. Unter den 7 Kindern mit posteriorer sagittaler Anorektoplastik fanden sich 4 Patienten, bei denen zusätzlich Elemente einer früheren Gracilis- oder Glutaeus-maximus-Plastik mit zur Rekonstruktion eines suffizienten Sphinkterapparates verwandt wurden. Von den 13 älteren Patienten mit sekundären kontinenzverbessernden Eingriffen wurden 7 vollständig kontinent, bei 6 Patienten wurde die Kontinenzleistung deutlich verbessert, so daß diese Kinder nun für festen und breiigen Stuhl kontinent sind, jedoch bei Streßsituationen und Diarrhö sowie gelegentlich nachts noch einschmieren. Kein Kind verblieb vollständig inkontinent.

Résumé

D'octobre 1984 à décembre 1986, 25 interventions dans le but d'améliorer une continence rectale ont été pratiquées à l'hôpital des enfants de Cologne. Chez 8 nourrissons, une plastie d'inversion a été réalisée dans le but de reconstituer un muscle abdomino-sacro-périnéal. Chez 4 nouveaux-

Paediatric Surgical Clinic, Children's Hospital of Cologne, Amsterdamerstrasse 59, D-5000 Köln 60, Federal Republic of Germany

Progress in Pediatric Surgery, Vol. 25
Angerpointner (Ed.)
© Springer-Verlag Berlin Heidelberg 1990

nés de sexe féminin, il fut pratiqué une plastie ano-rectale sagittale. Il a fallu réintervenir chez 13 patients: 5 fois pour une plastie rectale sagittale antérieure secondaire et 7 fois pour une plastie ano-rectale postérieure sagittale. Chez un garçon, il a fallu pratiquer une transposition de Gracili d'après Pickrell. Sur les 7 enfants ayant subi une plastie ano-rectale postérieure sagittale, 4 cas ont permis la réutilisation d'une plastie antérieure de Gracili ou de Glutaens pour reconstruire un sphincter. Parmi les 17 patients plus âgés, opérés en vue d'amélioration de leur continence, 7 furent un plein succès et 6 eurent une amélioration appréciable, à tel point que tous ces enfants sont dès lors continents, quel que soit le type de selles mais, quoi qu'en cas de stress et de diarrhée et parfois la nuit, ils présentent encore quelques fuites. Aucun enfant ne resta totalement incontinent.

Introduction

Posterior sagittal anorectoplasty is based on the "rectotomia posterior" for resection of rectal carcinoma, described by Kraske [12] in 1885. In this operation, pelvic floor structures were dissected medially to provide broad access to the tumour. This classic approach was used by Stephens [19] in 1953 for sacroperineal pull-through in low and intermediate forms of anal atresia and for closure of rectovaginal and rectourethral fistulae. Stephens published further work on this method in 1963 [20] and 1971 [21].

As far as surgical treatment of faecal incontinence is concerned, Parks and McPartlin [15] first employed the posterior approach in 1971 for posterior release with reconstruction and tightening of the puborectalis sling. For the first time, the posterior sagittal approach was used by Kiesewetter and Jeffereies [10] in 1981 as a secondary operation for treatment of faecal incontinence in patients who were operated on for anal atresia. They have already reported 10-year-results with their method which was also described by de Vries [3] in 1982 and Pena [17] in 1983. Kiesewetter and Jeffereis transected the pelvic floor structures, including the puborectalis sling in the median plane, and subsequently freed the anus from the perineum by means of a circular incision in order to expose puborectalis fibres at the dorsal wall of the urethra which would have been missed during abdominoperineal pull-through, and to sew them together dorsal to the rectum.

Thereafter the mobilized anorectum was reinserted into the perineum, taking into account the muscular sphincter structures. de Vries and Pena [3] and Pena [17] also used the posterior sagittal approach described by Kiesewetter for the correction of high anorectal atresias and cloacal malformations. Moreover, they underpinned their operative method by detailed embryological studies [1, 2, 16]. It has been shown, by the thorough investigations of Stephens [19] and the more recent anatomical studies of Huber et al. [7], that the primary sacral approach provides an excellent overview and a physiological reconstruction of the pelvic floor muscles in high and intermediate forms of anorectal atresia.

Since, however, pelvic floor and sphincter muscles may be hypoplastic in anorectal malformations (particularly in their high forms), the question arises how a secondary sacral reconstruction may contribute to improvement of faecal continence and what procedures may be employed if there are no usable muscular structures.

Table 1. Continence-improving operations performed at the Paediatric Surgical Clinic, Children's Hospital, Cologne, from October 1984 to December 1986

Patients, operation	Number
Neonates	
Smooth muscle inversion plasty	8
Anterior levator plasty	4
Other children	
Anterior levator plasty	5
Gracilis transposition	1
Posterior sagittal anorectoplasty with subsequent	7
Smooth muscle inversion plasty	3
Gracilis reconstruction	3
Gluteus maximus reconstruction	1
Total	25

Patients

From October 1984 to December 1986, 25 continence-improving operations were performed at the Paediatric Surgical Clinic of the Children's Hospital, Cologne (Table 1). Of these, 12 operations were carried out primarily in neonates; smooth muscle inversion plasties were employed during an abdominosacroperineal pull-through in 8 instances and anterior sagittal anorectoplasties (levator plasty) in 4 instances. Secondary continence-improving operations were performed in 13 children aged 4–19 years; anterior saggital anorectoplasties were applied in 5 patients, gracilis transposition according to Pickrell in 1 patient and secondary posterior sagittal anorectoplasties with additional smooth muscle sphincter plasty or simultaneous gracilis or gluteus maximus transposition in 7 patients. Operative techniques employed are briefly described separately or in the appropriate case reports.

Operative Techniques

Anterior Sagittal Anorectoplasty

Anterior sagittal anorectoplasty is based on the procedure described by Potts et al. [18] with circumcision of the rectovestibular fistula, detachment from the dorsal vagina and insertion into the centre of the perineal muscles. Additionally, the puborectalis muscles, the superficial transverse perineal muscles and, if present, the bulbocavernous muscles are adapted anterior to the newly created anal orifice. Thus, a robust perineum can be constructed and the muscles can be strengthened by adaptation of the striated muscle structures.

Posterior Sagittal Anorectoplasty

In posterior sagittal anorectoplasty, we follow the recommendations of Kiesewetter [8, 9], Kiesewetter and Jefferies [10] and de Vries and Pena [3, 17]. Since,
however, we found hypoplastic or scarry pelvic floor and puborectalis muscles
during the secondary continence-improving operations in three of seven patients,
for improvement of continence we employed Hofmann-von-Kap-herr's modification [6] of our smooth muscle inversion plasty described in 1981 [4, 5].

During the posterior sagittal approach we found rudimentary pelvic floor and
striated sphincter structures in four of seven children who had, however, partly
atrophied muscle transplants secondary to previous gracilis or gluteus maximus
transpositions. These were used for construction of an anal sphincter, briefly described in the following case reports:

Case 1. Date of birth 28 July 1975. Underwent an abdominoperineal pull-through
for high anorectal atresia with rectourethral fistula in 1976. This was followed by
right-sided gracilis transposition in 1981, but with the transposition around the
anus performed anticlockwise. The patient was entirely incontinent postoperatively. On posterior sagittal anorectoplasty performed in 1985, we found a gracilis
muscle sling originating from the right side and fading out at 9 o'clock, which was,
however, long enough to be fixed on the ipsilateral tuber ossis ischii. Moreover,
the patient had, dorsal to the anus a strong muscle structure which was slung
around the rectum distal to the gracilis muscle (Fig. 1a–d). Additionally, the
hypoplastic levator ani and puborectalis muscles were tightened.

Postoperatively, we found a marked increase of the anorectal pressure profile
and the voluntary pressure profile from 8 to 15 mm Hg and 25 to 35 mm Hg, respectively, as compared with preoperative values (Fig. 2a). On slowly withdraw-
ing the manometry catheter we recognized that the gracilis muscle contributed
more to continence than the distal muscle structures (Fig. 2b). After inflation with
20 ml physiological saline solution, high amplitude waves appeared owing to the
narrow and inelastic upper rectum after pull-through. This pressure increase felt
by the boy was answered by strong voluntary contractions, achieving control of
these high amplitude waves without defecation (Fig. 2c). There were rudimentary
relaxations during rest with overflow of a few drops of saline, answered by prompt
voluntary contractions. This behaviour corresponds to nearly normal continence
with slight soiling under stress and at night (Fig. 2d).

Case 2. Date of birth 9 March 1968. This girl sustained a severe car accident in
April 1973 with extended compound pelvic fracture, severe soft tissue injury of
the vagina and rectum, and complete destruction of the sphincter apparatus as
well as partial loss of the major labia. Treatment consisted of reduction of the
pelvic fracture with adaptation of the symphysis, osteosynthesis of the upper
pubic arch and reconstruction of rectum, vagina and labia. In 1974 gracilis transposition on the right side. From 1974 to 1983 electrostimulation of the gracilis
muscle without success. In 1983 reconstruction of the perineum and resection of a

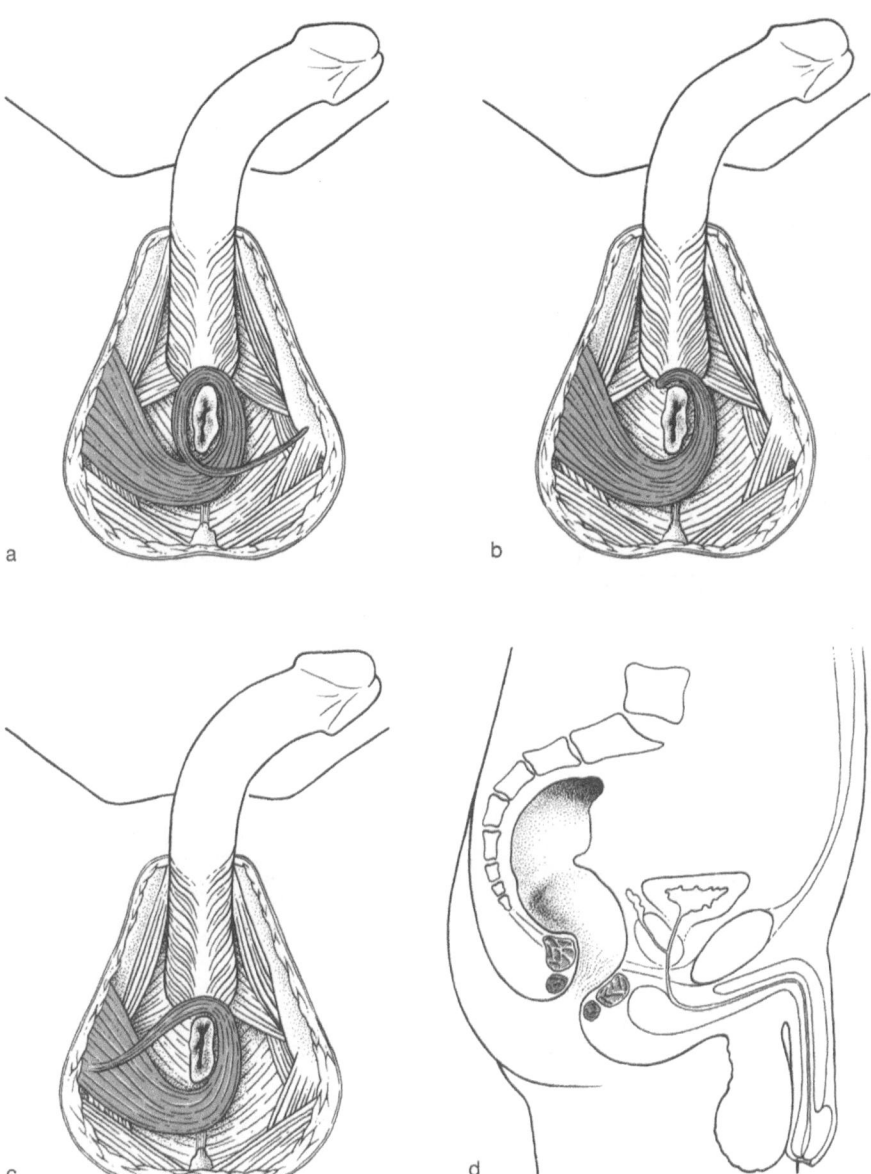

Fig. 1a–d. Case 1: High anorectal atresia, state after right-sided gracilis transposition. **a** Transposed gracilis muscle, slung around the anus from posterior to anterior, fading out at 9 o'clock, **b** fibrotic part of the gracilis muscle removed, **c** fixation of the gracilis muscle sling to the ipsilateral tuberculum ossis ischii, **d** sagittal section with exposure of the gracilis muscle sling and muscle structures distally readapted around the anal canal in a circular fashion

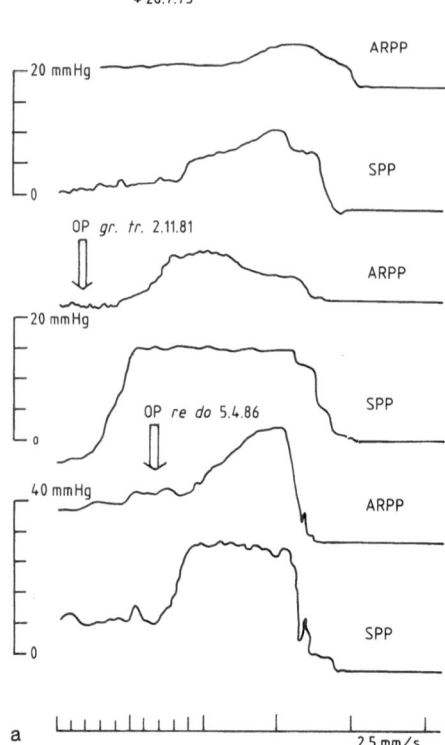

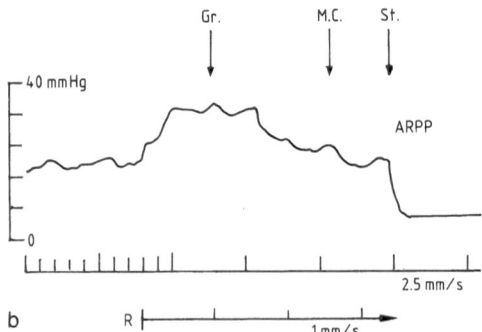

Fig. 2a, b

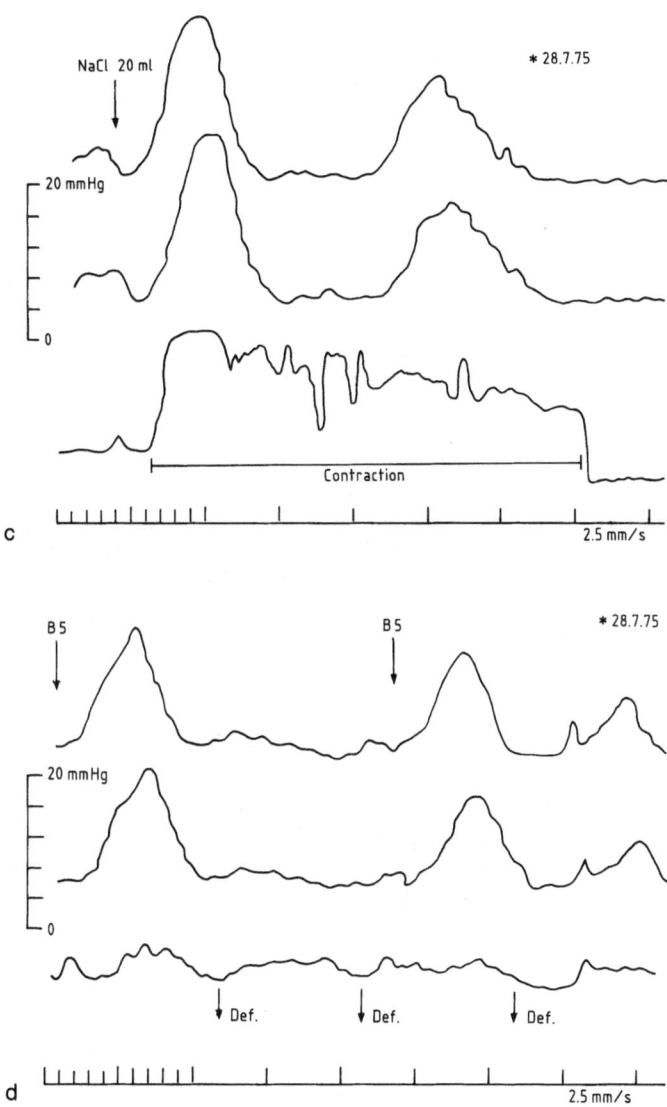

Fig. 2a–d. Case 1: Postoperative electromanometric findings. **a** Increase of the resting anorectal pressure profile *(ARPP)* and the voluntary contraction profile *(SPP)* prior to surgery *(top)*, secondary to gracilis transposition *(middle)* and posterior sagittal anorectoplasty *(bottom)*. Marked improvement of resting pressure as well as voluntary contraction profile, **b** resting pressure profile during slow withdrawal of the catheter from the anal canal: clear exposure of the gracilis muscle sling *(GR)*, the muscle structures *(M.C.)* and a slight scarry stenosis *(S.T.)* at the mucocutaneous junction, **c** high amplitude multisegmental waves following rectosigmoidal stimulation with 20 ml physiological saline. The waves can be halted by voluntary sphincter contraction, preventing defecation, **d** high amplitude multisegmental waves following rectal stimulation with 5 ml air by balloon. Rudimentary relaxations of the internal sphincter, associated with overflow of a few drops of bowel contents. Only low contraction peaks in the sense of a continence reaction

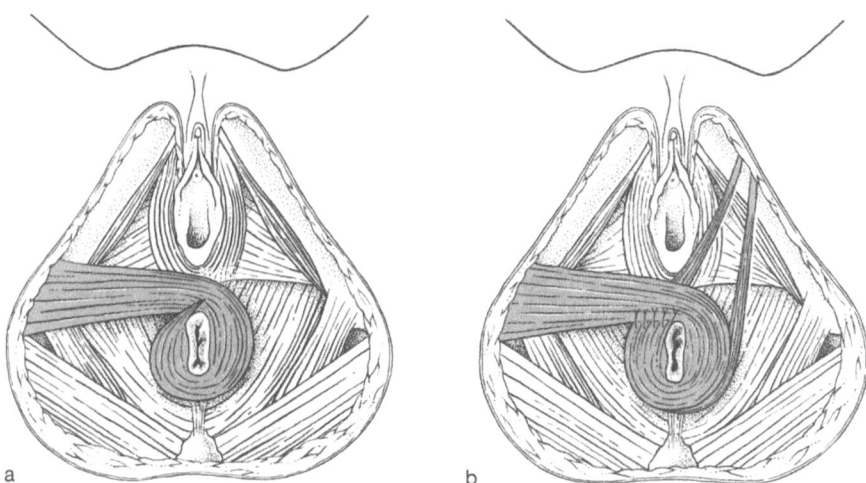

Fig. 3a, b. Case 2: State following car accident with traumatic impalement injury, gracilis transposition. **a** Semicircular muscle sling with fibrotic degeneration at 9 o'clock, **b** suturing of the gracilis muscles to each other and supportive palmaris longus transplantation

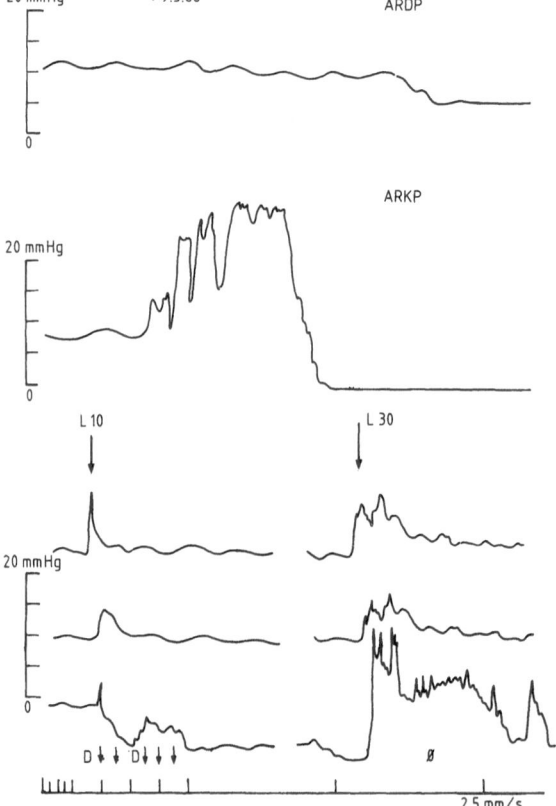

Fig. 4. Case 2: Electromagnometric follow-up, low anorectal resting pressure profile *(ARDP)*, vigorous anorectal contraction profile *(ARKP)*, rudimentary relaxations of the internal sphincter and weak voluntary contraction following inflation of 10 ml air into the rectosigmoid. Complete halt of overflow of air or saline by simultaneous voluntary contraction, i. e. good function of transposed and transplanted muscles

mucosal prolapse. Indication for posterior sagittal secondary anorectoplasty in 1985 for persistent incontinence. Since preoperative electrostimulation did not show the presence of contractile tissue, a palmaris longus transplantation was additionally prepared;14 days after denervation of the palmaris longus muscle the posterior sagittal secondary anorectoplasty was performed. The anal orifice was found outside the muscle apparatus which seemed to be rudimentary. There was only a semicircular sling of the gracilis muscle around the rectum, fading out at 9 o'clock.

There was not enough muscle for refixation at the ipsilateral tuberculum ossis ischii. Therefore, the remaining muscle was sutured to itself (Fig. 3a, b) and the palmaris longus transplantation was additionally carried out so that the palmaris longus tracts were brought into close contact with the pelvic floor proximal to the gracilis sling and fixed to the left lower pubic arch. Firm tightening thus provided a support against the contraction of the gracilis sling.

Postoperatively, there was a marked increase of the anorectal voluntary contraction profile from 12 mm Hg (preoperative value) to 30 mm Hg, whereas the resting pressure profile did not improve significantly (Fig. 4). As in our first patient, stimulation of the rectosigmoid with 10 ml air produced an overflow of a few drops of bowel contents, followed by prompt voluntary contraction. These defecations could be avoided by voluntary contractions of the newly created sphincter muscles. The girl is continent for solid and pultaceous stools. Only under stress or diarrhoea do signs of incontinence appear.

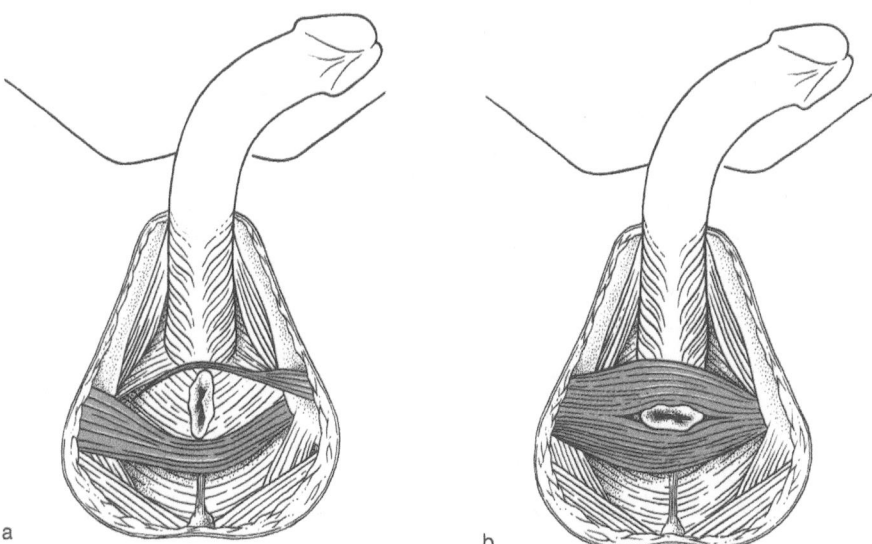

a   b

Fig. 5a, b. Case 4: State following high anorectal atresia with rectourethral fistula, abdominoperineal pull-through, gluteus maximus plasty according to Shoemaker. **a** Rudimentary anterior part of the gluteus maximus muscle. **b** State after pulling the mobilized anorectum through the bipartite muscle remnant

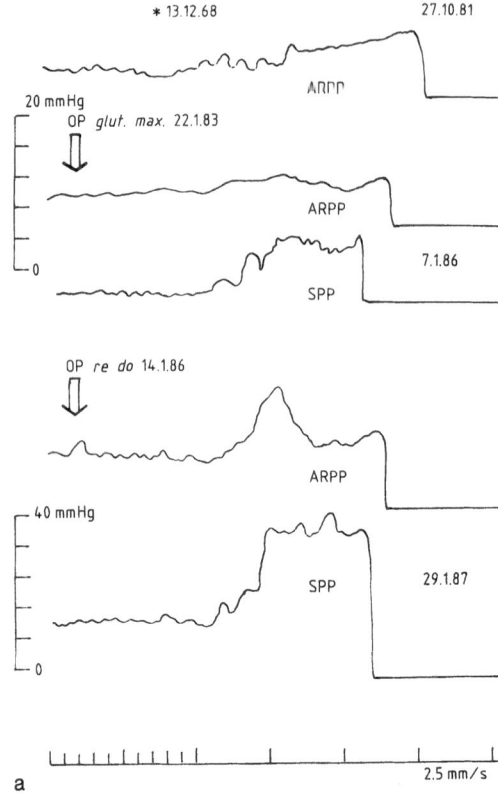

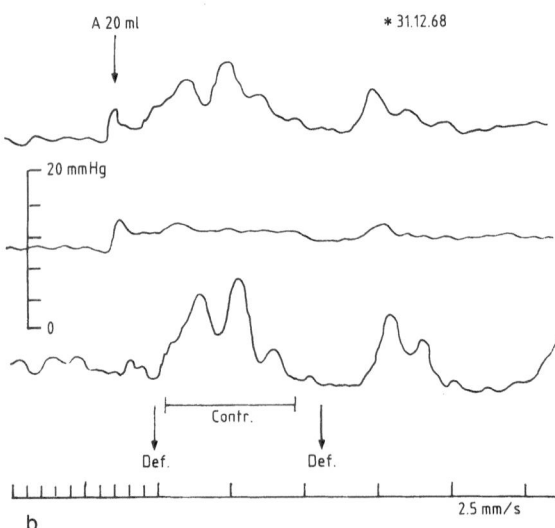

Fig. 6a, b

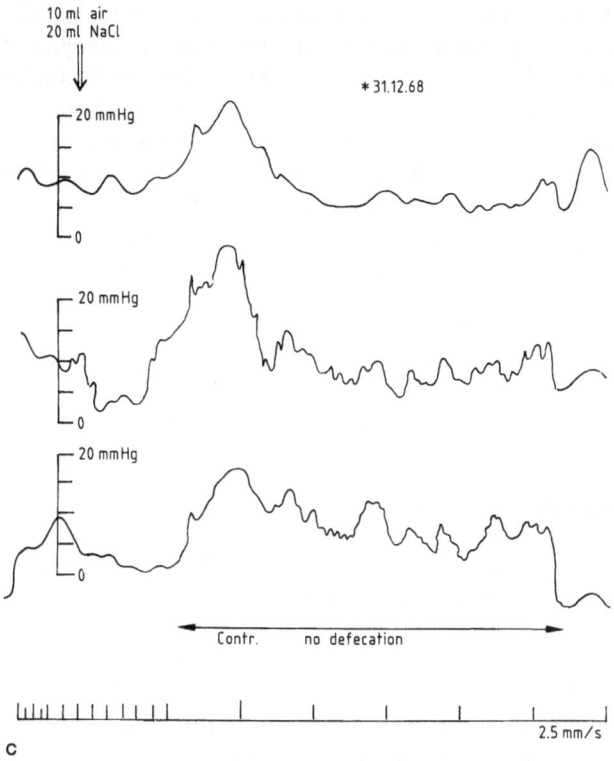

Fig. 6a–c. Case 4: Electromanometric follow-up. **a** Anorectal resting pressure profile *(ARPP)* and contraction profile *(SPP)* prior to gluteus maximus transposition *(top)*, thereafter *(middle)* and following posterior sagittal anorectoplasty *(bottom)*. Clear increase of resting and voluntary contraction profile, **b** rectosigmoidal stimulation with 20 ml air *(A)*, slight adaptation reaction in the rectum, inhibition of incipient defecation by voluntary contraction, **c** rectal stimulation with 10 ml air and 20 ml physiological saline. High amplitude multisegmental waves in the rectosigmoid, rectum and anorectum, but no defecation. Despite low rectal compliance, the waves can be fully compensated by voluntary contractions, providing full continence.

Case 3. We found a similar situation in a 12-year-old boy following high anorectal atresia and gracilis transposition. During posterior sagittal anorectoplasty, which became necessary because of complete incontinence, we found a strong gracilis sling which, however, faded out at 3 o'clock, leading to an incomplete and ineffective gracilis ring. We exposed the sling, tightened the gracilis muscle and fixed it to the contralateral tuberculum ossis ischii. Thereafter the muscle fibres were bluntly divided in the middle of the transplant and the anorectum was pulled through and fixed to the centre of the muscle structures. The boy showed full continence postoperatively.

Case 4. Date of birth 31 December 1968. An abdominoperineal pull-through was performed in 1970 in this boy for high anorectal atresia with rectourethral fistula.

In 1983 gluteus maximus plasty according to Shoemaker. Subsequently, three anal dilatation plasties and resection of mucosal ectopias. Persistent faecal incontinence. In 1986 secondary posterior sagittal anorectoplasty. During operation we found an atrophied perineal gluteus maximus flap, whereas the sacral flap was well maintained (Fig. 5a, b). We resected another recurrent rectal prolapse and (as in our previous case) pulled the rectum through the transversely separated strong part of the gluteus maximus muscle and sewed the hypoplastic muscle fibres together around the modelled anorectum. Postoperatively, the anorectal resting pressure profile and voluntary contraction profile increased markedly from 10 and 12 mm Hg to 20 and 40 mm Hg, respectively (Fig. 6a).

On stimulating the rectosigmoid with 20 ml air, discharge of air from the anus was immediately disrupted by strong contractions of the gluteus maximus muscle (Fig. 6b), likewise during instillation of physiological saline and air into the rectosigmoid (Fig. 6c). The boy is fully continent for solid and fluid stools as well as for flatus.

Results

Postoperatively, all 13 older children were reinvestigated clinically and electromanometrically after a minimum of 6 months. Four of five children who underwent anterior levator plasty were fully continent and the remaining patient showed considerably improved continence. This girl sustained a wound infection postoperatively, leading to stenosis. Bougienage treatment was unsuccessful, necessitating dilatation plasty according to Heinicke-von Mikulicz. The girl is continent, but exhibits soiling during stress and diarrhoea. The same is true of the boy with gracilis transposition who was entirely incontinent preoperatively; first-degree partial continence with slight soiling during stress and diarrhoea has been achieved.

Three of seven children became fully continent by means of posterior sagittal anorectoplasty, the remaining four achieved considerably improved continence

Table 2. Results in 13 children who underwent secondary continence-improving operations

Procedure	Patients	Continent	Clearly improved	In-continent	Complications
Anterior levator plasty	5	4	1		Wound infection + stricture ($n = 1$)
Gracilis transplantation	1		1		
Posterior sagittal anorectoplasty with subsequent					
Smooth muscle inversion	3	1	2		Stenoses ($n = 3$)
Gracilis reconstruction	3	1	2		Infection with stenosis ($n = 1$)
Gluteus maximus reconstruction	1	1			
Total	13	7	6		5

(Table 2). However, the three patients who had smooth muscle inversion plasty, according to Hofmann-von-Kap-herr developed anorectal stenoses necessitating long-term bougienage or dilatation plasty according to Heinicke-von Mikulicz.

One patient with gracilis reconstruction and fixation of the gracilis sling to the ipsilateral tuberculum ossis ischii and reconstruction of muscle structures sustained postoperative wound infection and retraction of the anal mucosa. A preternatural anus had to be established which was otherwise not the primary rule in posterior sagittal anorectoplasty. When the patient had overcome the infection the mucosa was reimplanted into the perineum. Dilatation treatment is still under way.

Two of four patients who had posterior sagittal anorectoplasty with additional gracilis or gluteus maximus reconstruction became fully continent and two achieved improved continence for solid and pultaceous stools. Of the 13 older children who had undergone secondary continence-improving operations, 7 achieved complete continence and 6 considerable improved continence. Napkins which were preoperatively worn by all 13 patients could be omitted postoperatively; 6 patients exhibit soiling under stress and diarrhoea.

Discussion

Our investigations show that muscle structures found during secondary posterior sagittal anorectoplasty are often insufficient for reconstruction of an external sphincter or efficient puborectalis sling. Both organs are not infrequently hypoplastic or cicatrized owing to previous abdominoperineal pull-through, as was the case in the three children in whom a smooth muscle sphincter plasty had to be performed in addition to posterior sagittal anorectoplasty, and in the four children with reconstruction of a strong muscle sling by means of remnants of the gracilis or gluteus maximus muscles.

In all patients a gaping anal orifice persisted, whereas the anal canal could be entirely closed by voluntary contractions. D'Guessan and Stephens [14] reported on a neonate with low anal atresia and subcutaneous fistula who died from multiple anomalies at the age of 18 days. Pathohistological findings confirmed our experience that muscle structures may contain only parts of a normal external profound anal sphincter and may be hypoplastic, even in low forms of anal atresia.

Our investigations further show that secondary reconstruction of the anorectum carries an increased risk of wound infection and that the excellent results observed by Pena and de Vries [2, 3, 16, 17] are by no means standard. Thus, Nakayama et al. (1986) reported 26 surgical complications which occurred despite colostomy. From 1982 to 1985 they performed posterior sagittal anorectoplasty in 23 patients and observed infections with retractions of vaginal and anal orifices, transitory femoralis nerve paralysis, suture insufficiency of the modelled rectum, rectourethral fistula, development of a posterior rectal diverticulum caused by insufficient support of the dorsal rectal wall by hypoplastic pelvic floor muscles as well as rectocutaneous fistulae and dehiscence of the sacroperineal incision.

Pena (1982) found 34 complications in 132 patients with primary and secondary posterior sagittal anorectoplasties, such as constipation ($n = 10$), mucosal prolapse ($n = 7$), diarrhoea ($n = 4$), anal stricture ($n = 6$), wound infection ($n = 2$), urethrovaginal fistula ($n = 2$) and postoperative urinary retention ($n = 3$). Kiesewetter and Jeffereies [10] reported in 1979 on their results of posterior sagittal anorectoplasty. Of 25 patients' 6 achieved normal continence (24%), 13 achieved socially acceptable continence (52%), defined as voluntary control of continence with occasional soiling, 4 children exhibited regular soiling (16%) and 2 remained incontinent (8%).

Kiesewetter's and Jeffereis' reports were long-term observations over 5–10 years, showing that 40% of their 25 patients became continent at puberty, indicating that initially hypoplastic pelvic floor structures can be reinforced by growth. These authors performed electromanometric measurements in 10 of their 25 patients: 2 children exhibited normal parameters, 5 a decreased puborectalis muscle tone not providing secure continence later on and the remaining children showed borderline results in accordance with our electromanometric and clinical results.

Pena [16] reported in 1985 on his results in 132 sacroperineal reconstructions, distinguishing, however, only between excellent results, defined as voluntary control of continence without soiling, and good results in children less than 3 years with 1–3 involuntary defecations per day without soiling. Moreover, he separated poor continence with permanent faecal incontinence and reflex defecation. He gave preliminary figures in 53 children with rectourethral fistulae, according to which 22 children exhibited excellent continence, 13 good continence and 2 poor continence; 10 children could not be reinvestigated and in 6 patients the colostomy was not yet closed. These results are in contrast to those described by Pena [17] in 1983, according to which five of the eight patients investigated were continent with voluntary control of defecation without soiling and three were on the one hand able to control defecation voluntarily, but on the other showed unrecognized, reflex defecations when playing (encopresis).

We have made similar observations and could achieve an improvement only by use of additional muscle structures. de Vries and Pena [3] reported on 12 patients, clinically assessed after closure of colostomy. Eight of these patients obtained excellent results with 2–4 defecations per day without soiling. In four patients results were unsatisfactory; additional sacral anomalies with impaired neuromuscular function were responsible for failure of operation in three children.

However, reasonable results can be achieved by other continence-improving procedures; the results are comparable to our experience with posterior sagittal anorectoplasty. For instance, a series recently published by Kottmeier et al. [11] may be mentioned, according to which 8 of 18 patients with high anorectal atresia who had undergone levator mobilization and tightening (a procedure developed by the authors) achieved continence and 6 marked improvement of continence; only 4 patients remained incontinent. Therefore, the question arises to what effect the observed improvement of continence following posterior sagittal anorectoplasty can really be attributed: the incorporation of the muscle complex into the sphincter, the tightening of pelvic floor and puborectalis muscles after transection, the restoration of the anorectal angle by junction of the muscle stumps or modelling of the rectum (which is, however, unnecessary according to de Vries, in contrast to Pena). Our experience shows that complete success can only be achieved if there is sufficient muscle material for sphincter replacement, no neurogenic bladder or voiding disturbances are present and no infections occur postoperatively. For that reason, posterior sagittal anorectoplasty should be performed only under a protective colostomy. One should not be discouraged by previous unsuccessful gracilis or gluteus maximus transposition which can be integrated into the concept of posterior sagittal anorectoplasty.

References

1. de Vries PA (1984) The surgery of anorectal anomalies: its evolution with evaluation of procedures. Curr Probl Surg 21:1–75
2. de Vries PA, Cox KL (1985) Surgery of anorectal anomalies. Surg Clin North Am 65:1139–1169
3. de Vries PA, Pena A (1982) Posterior sagittal anorectoplasty. J Pediatr Surg 17:638–643
4. Holschneider AM, Hecker WC (1981) Gestielte und freie Muskeltransplantationen zur Behandlung der Stuhlinkontinenz. Z Kinderchir 32:244–258
5. Holschneider AM, Hecker WC (1981) Smooth muscle plasty: a new method of treating anorectal incontinence in infants with high anal and rectal atresia. J Pediatr Surg 16:917–920
6. Hofmann-von-Kap-herr S, Koltai JL (1983) Die glattmuskuläre Umstülpplastik mit Halbzylinderdoppelung. In: Hofmann-von-Kap-herr S (ed) Anorektale Fehlbildungen. Fischer, Stuttgart
7. Huber A, von Hochstetter AHC, Allgöver M (1983) Transsphinktere Rektumchirurgie. Topographische Anatomie und Operationstechnik. Springer, Berlin Heidelberg New York Tokio
8. Kiesewetter WB (1979) Rectum and anus. In: Ravitch MM, Welch KJ, Benson CD, et al (eds) Pediatric Surgery. Year Book, Medical Publishers, Chicago, p 1069
9. Kiesewetter WB (1980) Imperforate anus. In: Holder T, Ashcraft KW (eds) Pediatric Surgery. Saunders, Philadelphia, pp 412–413
10. Kiesewetter WB, Jeffereis MR (1981) Secondary anorectal surgery for the missed puborectalis muscle. J Pediatr Surg 16:921–926
11. Kottmeier PK, Veltek FT, Klotz DH, Coren CV, Hansbrough F, Price AP (1986) Results of levator plasty for anal incontinence. J Pediatr Surg 21:647–659
12. Kraske P (1885) Zur Exstirpation hochsitzender Mastdarm-Krebse. Verh Dtsch Ges Chir 14:464
13. Nakayama DK, Templeton JM, Ziegler MM, O'Neil JA, Walker AB (1986) Complications of posterior sagittal anorectoplasty. J Pediatr Surg 21:488–492
14. D'Guessan G, Stephens FD (1986) Covered anus with anocutaneous fistula: the muscular sphincters. J Pediatr Surg 21:33–35
15. Parks AG, McPartlin JF (1971) Late repair of injuries of the anal sphincter. Proc R Soc Med 64:1187
16. Pena A (1985) Surgical treatment of high imperforate anus. World J Surg 9:936–943
17. Pena A (1983) Posterior sagittal anorectal plasty as a secondary operation for the treatment of fecal incontinence. J Pediatr Surg 18:762–773
18. Potts WJ, Ricker WL, De Boer A (1954) Imperforate anus with recto vesical, recto urethral, recto vaginal and recto perineal fistula. Ann Surg 140:381
19. Stephens FD (1953) Imperforate rectum. A new surgical technique. Med J Aust 1:202
20. Stephens FD (1963) Congenital malformations of the rectum, anus and genito-urinary tract. Livingstone, Edinbourgh
21. Stephens FD, Smith EP (1971) Anorectal malformations in children. Year Book Medical Publishers, Chicago

Total Correction of Complete Atrioventricular Canal: Surgical Technique and Analysis of Long-Term Results

A. E. Urban

Summary

Surgery for total correction of complete AVC can be done with low early and late mortality. The operative risk is high only in patients who reach the operating room in a near moribund condition (NYHA V). There is clinical evidence that early operation – before the onset of pulmonary vascular disease – will further lower early and late mortality. The surgical technique has been refined to avoid late reoperation for left atrioventricular valve incompetence. The early and late results of operative therapy compare favourably with the natural history of this complex congenital cardiac disease.

Zusammenfassung

Die operative Behandlung des kompletten AV-Kanals kann mit niedriger Früh- und Spätletalität durchgeführt werden. Das Operationsrisiko ist nur bei den Patienten hoch, die den OP in nahezu moribundem Zustand erreichen. Klinische Erfahrungen zeigen, daß eine frühe Operation – vor Einsetzen einer pulmonalen Gefäßkrankheit – die Früh- und Spätletalität weiter senkt. Die chirurgische Technik wurde soweit verfeinert, daß eine Spätoperation wegen Insuffizienz der linken AV-Klappe vermieden wird. Früh- und Spätergebnisse sind günstig im Vergleich zum natürlichen Verlauf dieses höchst komplexen kongenitalen Vitiums.

Résumé

L'opération pour corriger le canal atrio-venticulaire peut être effectueé avec un taux de mortalité précoce et tardive relativement bas. Le risque opératoire est important uniquement dans les cas moribonds pré-opératoires. Les données cliniques démontrent que, l'opération étant réaliseé le plus tôt possible, c.ã.d, avant l'apparition d'une hypertension pulmonaire, le taux de mortalité precoce et tardive en est d'autant plus bas. La technique opératoire a êté perfectionneé ã un tel point qu'elle permet d'éviter une éventuelle réoperation ã cause d'un fonctionnement insuffisant de la valve gauche atrio-ventriculaire. Les résultats obtenus ã court et ã long terme montrent, en comparaison avec l'evolution naturelle de cette maladie congenitale trés complexe, les avantages de l'intervention chirurgicale.

Introduction

Successful correction of the complete form of atrioventricular (septal) canal (AVC) defect is now readily achievable and has favourably altered the natural history of the disease. Without surgery 80% of patients die in the first 2 years of life [1].

Department of Cardiothoracic Surgery, Johanniter-Kinderklinik, Arnold-Janssen-Strasse 29, D-5205 Sankt Augustin, Federal Republic of Germany

Progress in Pediatric Surgery, Vol. 25
Angerpointner (Ed.)
© Springer-Verlag Berlin Heidelberg 1990

Patients and Methods

In 1981 we introduced the "two-patch, three-leaflet" [2] concept for total correction of AVC [3] in our unit. To date 88 consecutive patients have been operated on; 40 (45.5%) were female and 48 (54.5%) were male, 51 (58%) had Down's syndrome. The age ranged between 7 weeks and 138 months, 35 patients were under the age of 1 year, 25 under the age of 2 years and 28 were older. Their weight ranged between 2.4 and 21.7 kg (mean 9.2 kg).

In all, 75 patients (85.2%) had the complete form of AVC with large interventricular communication (VSD), 13 patients (14.7%) had intermediate AVC [4] with haemodynamically insignificant VSD. All survivors were traced for follow-up at 6–82 months (mean 34.1 months). A total of 21 operative procedures had been performed in 12 patients prior to total correction. These included division of patent ductus arteriosus (9 cases), lung biopsy (7), pulmonary artery banding (4) and attempted repair in another institution (1). Some 59 associated cardiac anomalies were corrected in 35 patients at the time of definite repair. These included ligation of patent ductus arteriosus (19), closure of atrial septal defect other than the primum defect or patent foramen ovale (17), correction of multiple VSDs (11), Fallot's tetralogy (4) and repair of other complex intracardiac malformations (8).

Operative Technique

Surgery is conducted with conventional cardiopulmonary bypass, direct cannulation of both vv. cavae and deep hypothermic reduced flow in the infants. Myocardial protection consist of cold cardioplegic solution and topical hypothermia. After the right atrium is opened, iced saline is injected to close the leaflets of the common atrioventricular valve and a stay suture placed at the most septal point where the left superior and left inferior bridging leaflets coapt. An appropriately tailored Dacron patch is then sutured in place with 4–0 or 5–0 interrupted sutures to close the ventricular part of the common atrioventricular septal defect.

The glutaraldehyde-preserved autologous pericardial patch is now inserted. It is sutured to the Dacron patch with interrupted 6–0 polypropylene sutures, which catch the two superior and inferior bridging leaflets, sandwiching them securely between the two patches. As a modification of the original technique applied in the last 11 patients, an appropriately sized Hegar is passed through the left atrioventricular valve component and the "cleft" closed by approximating the left superior and left inferior bridging leaflets with 6–0 interrupted polypropylene sutures, thus avoiding any stenosis. An anuloplasty is usually not necessary and is not done routinely.

The pericardial patch is then sutured in place to close the atrial component of the complete atrioventricular septal defect. This is done with a 6–0 or 5–0 polypropylene running suture, leaving the coronary sinus draining to the left atrium, thus minimizing the risk of heart block. Atrial and ventricular pacemaker wires are inserted, and left atrial and pulmonary artery catheters for postoperative pressure monitoring are placed routinely in all patients. The postoperative care is as usual; if pulmonary hypertensive episodes occur, they are treated according to protocol.

Methods of Analysis

For statistical analysis we used Fisher's exact test for 2 × 2 tables and Wilcoxson's test for comparison of survival times. We considered a statistical difference significant if the P value was 0.05 or smaller and if the 70% confidence limits (C.L.) were not overlapping. Potential risk factors for hospital death and premature late death were determined univariately.

As potential risk factors for hospital death, we investigated: age, weight, weight percentile, preoperative condition, year of operation, associated cardiac anomalies, previous cardiac operations, morphology of the bridging leaflets, type of atrioventricular septal defect with its size and relation to the bridging leaflets, and the degree of preoperative atrioventricular valve incompetence.

Results

Of the 88 patients, 5 (5.7%, 70% C.L. 3.2%–9.7%) died in hospital (30-day mortality) and 8 (9.1%) died late with an overall mortality of 13 (14.8%). There was no early or premature late death in the 8 patients who required reoperation for atrioventricular valve repair failure. No patient (0%, 70%, C.L. 0%–2.15%) developed complete heart block. Modes of early death included acute cardiac failure in 3 and pulmonary hypertensive episodes in 2. Causes of late death were pulmonary vascular disease with acute right heart failure in 4, left atrioventricular valve incompetence in 3 and a noncardiac accident in 1.

Of 83 early survivors, 8 (9.6%) required reoperations for incompetence of the left atrioventricular valve 2 days to 26 months after the initial repair. If the repair failed owing to dehiscense of the valve leaflets from the patch this usually occurred early, in a matter of days or weeks. If the incompetence was to be reoperated on late, it was usually through the "cleft" between the anterior and posterior bridging leaflets. The procedures were in keeping with this mode of incompetence. There were three left atrioventricular valve replacements and five reconstructions of the mitral valve component, mainly by adapting the two bridging leaflets and thus closing the "cleft". Valvuloplasties were necessary in two cases to achieve a smaller valve ring.

Younger age at repair, earlier date of operation, lower weight at the time of total correction and lower weight percentile were not incremental risk factors for early and premature late death (Table 1). There were no deaths in 11 patients operated in the first 6 months of life. The presence of major associated cardiac anomalies had no bearing on the outcome of the operation (Table 2). There was no mortality in 4 patients with additional Fallot's tetralogy, in 2 patients with double outlet right ventricle and pulmonary stenosis or in 11 patients with multiple ventricular septal defects.

Table 1. Hospital death related to age at repair

Age (months)	No.	Died	%	70% C.L.
0– 6	11	0	0	0 –15.84
6– 12	23	3	13.0	6.14–25.49
12– 48	35	2	5.71	1.96–12.97
48–138	19	0	0	0 – 9.5

C.L. confidence limits

Table 2. Hospital death related to presence of major associated cardiac anomalies

Anomaly	No.	Died	%	70% C.L.
Fallot's tetralogy	4	0	0	0–37.76
DORV + PS	2	0	0	0–61.27
VSD mult.	11	0	0	0–15.84

C.L. confidence limits; DORV + PS double-outlet right ventricle and pulmonary stenosis; VSD mult. multiple ventricular septal defects

The only significant ($P = 0.025$) risk factor for hospital death was a preoperative functional class V (New York Heart Association, NYHA). Of the 83 patients in NYHA classes II–IV, 3 died in hospital (3.6%, 70% C.L. 1.6%–7.2%); of the 5 in NYHA class V, 2 died (40%, 70% C.L. 24.2%–71%).

More severe preoperative atrioventricular valve incompetence did not increase the risk of early or premature late death. Of the 42 patients with absent to mild atrioventricular valve incompetence 3 died (7.14%, 70% C.L. 3.19%–13.81%) and of the 32 patients with moderate to severe incompetence 2 died (6.25%, 70% C.L. 2.14%–14.14%). Patients in whom the degree of preoperative atrioventricular valve incompetence could not be stated exactly were not included in this calculation.

On the other hand, more severe preoperative atrioventricular valve incompetence was the only significant ($P = 0.005$) incremental risk factor for reoperation. None of the 42 patients with absent to mild atrioventricular valve incompetence needed reoperation (0%, 70% C.L. 0%–4.4%) whereas 6 of the 32 patients with more severe preoperative valve incompetence had to be reoperated for valve repair failure (18.8%, 70% C.L. 11.4%–28.4%). The 14 patients (2 reoperations) for whom there was incomplete knowledge of the preoperative severity of their left atrioventricular valve incompetence were again excluded from this evaluation.

Discussion

Only two incremental risk factors – the preoperative functional status for early death and a more severe preoperative left atrioventricular valve incompetence for late reoperations – have evolved from the analysis of our data.

Yet operative and clinical experience tells us that there are remaining problems. The figure for post-repair left atrioventricular valve incompetence is important, 10% of the patients requiring reoperations with either reconstruction (5) or replacement (3) of the mitral component of the atrioventricular valve. Since 1987 we have therefore initiated a new approach to avoid this problem. Our intraoperative impression, substantiated by our findings at reoperation, is that in cases with no good chordal support of the bridging leaflets, leaving the "cleft" open will lead to late atrioventricular valve incompetence. We now therefore systematically close the "cleft" in all cases, providing this would not produce a stenotic valve, which in our experience should be the case only in double-orifice left atrioventricular valve and severe right ventricular dominance.

To date there is insufficient statistical support, even though none of the patients treated with this approach have developed any degree of late valve incompetence. This could possibly be due to the still small number of patients treated and the short follow-up. We therefore intend to continue on this line, hoping to be able to provide more evidence in the near future.

From analysis of age as a risk factor, it was clear that even a very young age at operation does not increase the probability of early death. Interestingly, all the early deaths are concentrated in an age group ranging from 6 to 48 months. In the first 6 months it is unlikely that an infant has already developed pulmonary vascular disease. After 48 months the population is selected for patients not at risk of pulmonary vascular disease.

There is convincing clinical evidence that pulmonary vascular disease could be one of the important determinants for early death at present. Because of the paucity of measurements available, the level of pulmonary vascular resistance could not be analysed. Still, this is the hypothesis on which we intend to work in the immediate future.

Acknowledgments. We thank Dr. R. Fimmers from the Institut für Statistik, Dokumentation und Datenverarbeitung der Universität Bonn for the statistical analysis.

References

1. Berger TJ, Blackstone EH, Kirklin JW, Bargeron LM, Hazelrig JB, Turner ME (1979) Survival and probability of cure without and with surgery in complete atrioventricular canal. Ann Thorac Surg 27:104
2. Carpentier A (1978) Surgical anatomy and management of the mitral component of atrioventricular canal defects. In: Anderson RH, Shinebourne EA (eds) Pediatric cardiology. Churchill Livingstone, London
3. Studer M, Blackstone EH, Kirklin JW, et al (1982) Determinants of early and late results of repair of atrioventricular septal (canal) defects. J Thorac Cardiovasc Surg 84:523–542
4. Becker AE, Anderson RH (1981) Pathology of congenital heart disease. Butterworths, London, pp 77–92

Nonosseous Lesions of the Anterior Cruciate Ligaments in Childhood and Adolescence

R. Kellenberger[2] and L. von Laer[1]

Summary

Damage of the knee joint has increased during the last few years owing to overindulgence in sports. The anterior cruciate ligaments play a major role in knee joint stability. Treatment of injured knee joint structures in childhood and adolescence is more complicated than in adults. From 1972 to 1987 we have seen 330 patients with knee injuries, 28 of whom had nonosseous lesions of the anterior curciate ligaments. Of these, 20 were followed-up; 17 children were operated on primarily, 3 were conservatively immobilized. On follow-up, 15 patients showed signs of residual instability. Primary treatment depends on the presence and the extent of associated injuries of the knee joint.

Zusammenfassung

Durch exzessiv betriebenen Sport nahmen die Kniegelenkverletzungen in den letzten Jahren zu. Die vorderen Kreuzbänder spielen für die Kniegelenkstabilität eine wichtige Rolle. Die Behandlung verletzter Kniegelenkbinnenstrukturen im Wachstumsalter ist komplizierter als beim Erwachsenen. 1972–1987 behandelten die Autoren 330 Kinder und Jugendliche mit Kniegelenkverletzungen, 28 davon mit nichtossären Läsionen der vorderen Kreuzbänder; 20 von ihnen konnten nachuntersucht werden. 17 Kinder waren primär operativ und 3 konservativ durch Ruhigstellung behandelt worden. Bei der Nachuntersuchung zeigten 15 Patienten Zeichen verbliebener Instabilität. Die primäre Behandlung hängt vom Vorhandensein und Ausmaß begleitender Kniegelenkverletzungen ab.

Résumé

Suite à une pratique excessive du sport, les lésions de l'articulation du genou augmentent. Les ligaments croisés antérieurs jouent un rôle capital dans la stabilité du genou. Le traitement des blessures intra-articulaires du genou durant la croissance représente une complication thérapeutique supérieure à celles des patients d'âge adulte. De 1972 à 1987, nous avons examiné 300 enfants et adolescents présentant des lésions du genou, dont 28 avec des lésions non-osseuses des ligaments croisés antérieurs. 20 ont pu être suivis. 17 enfants avaient été opérés et 3 immobilisés par un traitement conservateur. 15 patients continuaient à présenter par la suite une certaine instabilité. Le traitement initial doit être choisi en fonction des autres lésions de l'articulation du genou présentes et de leur gravité.

---

[1]Division of Traumatology and Division of Orthopaedics, Childrens Hospital of Basle, Römergasse 8, CH-4005 Basel, Switzerland
[2]Present address: Service de Chirurgie Orthopédique, Hôpital Cantonal, 1700 Fribourg, Switzerland

Introduction

Increasingly intensive sports, as well as new "safety" devices (e.g. ski bindings, ski boots) have led to a considerable and real rise in knee joint injuries which are not an artifact of improved diagnosis [32]. Damage primarily affects the anterior cruciate ligaments as central determinants of knee joint stability. In adult orthopaedics, the simple suture soon turned out to be sufficient [7, 9, 23, 29, 33]. Therefore, lesions of the cruciate ligaments in adults are treated primarily by ligament reconstruction with increasing frequency [7, 11, 13, 18]. Today aftercare is carried out functionally [12]. However, the number of recommended operative techniques as well as unsatisfactory results in 20%–30% of cases call into question whether complete recovery of stability is possible by surgical treatment alone [7, 11, 13, 14, 17, 18, 20, 21, 25, 27, 28, 31, 34, 36, 39].

We have also seen an increase of these injuries in children and adolescents. Treatment is more difficult in adolescents; diagnosis and therapy is simpler in children under 12 years of age. As in other skeletal parts, periosteal, chondral and osseous avulsions occur in 80% of cases up the the 12th year of age, whereas the ligaments remain intact or merely stretched. In knee injuries we find osseous avulsions of the anterior cruciate ligaments in 80% of cases, in the form of fractures of the intercondylar eminence of the tibia [1, 5, 22, 37]. Therefore, the prognosis depends less on problems of instability, but more on associated injuries, disturbances of growth and function as well as on pseudarthrosis. Beyond the 12th year of life, however, intraligamentous ruptures are increasingly observed, as in adults. Their treatment is more difficult than in adults as long as epiphyseal cartilages are still open. In contrast to eminence avulsions, the prognosis depends above all (as in adults) on problems of instability and their compensation, as well as on associated damage. There is only sparse literature on lesions of the anterior cruciate ligaments, predominantly on nonosseous lesions and their treatment in children and adolescents [3, 6, 8, 16, 18, 23, 33].

Analogous to the situation in adults, in the last few years we have employed with increasing frequency immediate diagnosis and operative repair of injured cruciate ligaments in adolescents. We have followed up our patients in order to achieve differential diagnosis and to clarify the question whether our procedure meets the demands of childhood and adolescence.

Patients

During the years 1972–1987 we have seen a total of 330 patients with knee injuries who presented primarily with haemarthrosis. We found 128 patients with primarily radiologically visible lesions (52 patella fractures, 35 eminence avulsions, 33 epiphysiolyses of the distal femur and 3 of the proximal tibia, 3 tibial tuberosity avulsions, 2 transitional fractures of the distal femoral epiphysis). In 155 patients a patella luxation could be diagnosed either anamnestically, clinically or radiologically. Isolated or combined interior knee joint injuries were found in 32 instances,

28 of them with lesions of the cruciate ligaments and 4 with isolated meniscus lesions. In 14 patients the cause of haemarthrosis remained unclear. Consequently, there were a total of 63 lesions of the cruciate ligaments, 35 of them osseous lesions (34 eminence avulsions, 1 posterior osseous cruciate ligament avulsion) and 28 nonosseous lesions. Age was less than 12 years in 80% of the patients with eminence avulsions ($n = 27$) and over 12 years in 90% of the patients with nonosseous lesions ($n = 25$). In this paper's classification, treatment and prognosis of eminence avulsion are not discussed, since our patients had been followed up in 1982 and 1987 and the results have been published elsewhere [37]. Our proposed classification into undislocated or incompletely dislocated avulsions which are conservatively treated, and completely dislocated avulsions which must be surgically treated has been confirmed by clinical application and follow-up.

Methods

Of the 28 patients with nonosseous lesions of the cruciate ligaments, 20 were clinically followed up in 1987 with a mean follow-up time of 4.3 years. Above all, we searched for recurrent knee joint effusions, swellings, pains and giving way as signs of instability. Moreover, we looked for blockages, pseudoblockages and the extent of sports activity before and after treatment.

Clinical investigations included the examination of the function of hip joint, knee joint and ankle joint, capsule swellings, effusions and differences of thigh circumference as possible signs of atrophy. Stability of the anterior cruciate ligament was studied using the anterior drawer test in 80° flexion, the Lachmann drawer sign, and the pivot shift sign, and the stability of the lateral ligaments was additionally examined according to a standardized medical examination form.

Results

Table 1 summarizes the results. The anterior cruciate ligaments were always affected in nonosseous lesions. There were a total of 5 periosteal avulsions (3 proximal, 2 distal) and 15 intraligamentous ruptures (2 partial ruptures, 13 complete ruptures). Types of lesions and distribution in patients with open and closed epiphyseal cartilages at the time of injury as well as isolated and combined lesions are shown in Table 2.

A total of 12 patients sustained combined injuries which are shown in Table 3. The combination of individual injuries can be seen in Table 1. Treatment employed is shown in Table 4. A total of 17 patients were treated surgically, 3 conservatively with cast immobilization. In recent years diagnosis was always made by arthroscopy, formerly by arthrotomy when corresponding clinical signs were present.

The follow-up results are shown in Tables 1 and 5. We found in 15 patients a positive Lachmann (drawer) sign in comparison with the contralateral side as a

Table 1. Nonosseous lesions of the cruciate ligaments in children and adolescents

Case	Age at accident (years)	State of epiphyseal cartilage	Associated damage	Treatment	Type of damage	In-stability	Follow-up data		
							Atrophy	Functional deficiency	Stability
1	8	Open	None	Conservative	Distal avulsion	Yes	No	No	Lachmann +
2	15	Premature	Medial collateral ligament, medial meniscus	Suture	Rupture	No	Yes	No	Lachmann +
3	14	Premature	None	Reinsertion	Proximal avulsion	Yes	Yes	No	Lachmann +
4	13	Open	Medial meniscus	Reinsertion	Proximal avulsion	No	No	No	Stable
5	13	Open	Posteromedial capsule triangle	Conservative	Partial rupture	No	No	No	Stable
6	15	Open	None	Conservative	Partial rupture	No	No	No	Stable
7	15	Open	Lateral collateral ligament, flake fracture	Suture	Rupture	No	No	No	Stable
8	13	Open	None	Suture	Rupture	No	Yes	No	Lachmann +
9	15	Open	Medial collateral ligament	Reinsertion	Proximal avulsion	No	No	No	Lachmann +
10	11	Open	Medial collateral ligament	Suture	Rupture	No	No	No	Lachmann +
11	16	Closed	None	Syndesmoplasty	Rupture	Yes	Yes	No	Lachmann +, pivot shift +
12	16	Closed	Posteromedial capsule triangle	Syndesmoplasty	Rupture	Yes	Yes	No	Lachmann +
13	17	Closed	Medial collateral ligament	Syndesmoplasty	Rupture	No	Yes	No	Lachmann +
14	16	Closed	None	Syndesmoplasty	Partial rupture	Yes	Yes	Yes	Lachmann +
15	18.	Closed	Cartilage	Suture	Rupture	No	Yes	No	Lachmann +
16	16	Closed	Lateral collateral ligament, lateral meniscus, postero-medial capsule triangle	Syndesmoplasty	Rupture	No	No	No	Lachmann +
17	14	Closed	Lateral meniscus, cartilage	Syndesmoplasty	Rupture	Yes	Yes	No	Lachmann +
18	14	Closed	Medial meniscus, cartilage	Syndesmoplasty	Rupture	No	No	No	Lachmann +
19	16	Closed	Lateral meniscus, medial collateral ligament	Reinsertion	Distal avulsion	Yes	Yes	No	Lachmann +
20	14	Closed	Medial meniscus, medial collateral ligament	Suture	Rupture	Yes	No	No	Stable

Table 2. Types of lesions

Lesion	Patients with open epiphyseal cartilage ($n = 10$)	Patients with closed epiphyseal cartilage ($n = 10$)
Avulsion ($n = 5$)	4	1
Rupture ($n = 13$)	5	8
Partial rupture ($n = 2$)	1	1
Isolated injury ($n = 8$)	4	4
Combined injury ($n = 12$)	6	6

Table 3. Associated lesions in 12 patients

Medial collateral ligament	6
Posteromedial capsule triangle	3
Medial meniscus	4
Lateral meniscus	3
Lateral collateral ligament	2
Cartilaginous damage	4

Table 4. Treatment

Treatment	Partial rupture ($n = 2$)	Avulsion ($n = 5$)	Rupture ($n = 13$)
A. *Surgical* ($n = 17$)			
Ligament reconstruction ($n = 7$)	1		6
Suture ($n = 6$)			6
Reinsertion ($n = 4$)		4	
B. *Conservative* ($n = 3$)	1	1	1

Table 5. Results

Positive Lachmann sign	15	(1 with additional pivot shift)
Pivot shift	1	
Instability anamnesis	8	(7 with positive Lachmann sign)
Quadriceps atrophy	10	(all with positive Lachmann sign)
Instability anamnesis plus quadriceps atrophy	6	(all with positive Lachmann sign)

sign of remaining instability. Six of these patients showed discrete symptoms of decompensation without effusions, but with limited ability to take part in sports; five of them occurred following ligament reconstruction and one following suture of a ruptured ligament. One patient presented with an anterior rotational instability with positive pivot shift sign, positive Lachmann sign, recurrent swellings, recurrent pain and limited ability to take part in sports. A positive Lachmann sign was found in all three conservatively treated patients, in three of four patients following reinsertion, in four of six patients following ligamentous sutures and in all seven patients following ligament reconstruction.

Two patients who had lost their cruciate ligaments (as shown via arthrotomy and secondary arthroscopy) developed an increasing knee joint stabilization during a follow-up of up to 10 years despite the absence of cruciate ligaments. This occurred in one case following suture of a ligamentous rupture and once following conservative treatment of a slightly dislocated, distal avulsion with a fine osseous lamella which had been primarily overlooked.

Discussion

The number of followed up cases with nonosseous lesions of the cruciate ligaments, the variability of treatment and the mostly short follow-up time do not allow a clear answer to the problems in question. There are only sporadic reports on lesions of the cruciate ligaments up to the 16th year of age in the literature [3, 5, 6, 8, 16, 19, 24, 38] which, moreover, mostly deal with eminence avulsions, thus being of little help in the assessment of nonosseous lesions of the cruciate ligaments. The remaining few patients with nonosseous lesions are not differentiated according to open or closed epiphyseal cartilages. There is no report of long-term follow-up on results of therapy which is mostly adapted from adult treatment and thus no statements on late prognosis.

Initially it was tried in adults to treat intraligamentous ruptures not only by augmentation plasty, but also primarily by autologous or homologous cruciate ligament transplantation, independent of associated damage, since better results seemed to be obtainable as compared with secondary treatment of knee joint instability [2, 4, 9, 11, 13, 18, 23, 25]. However, it was assumed that every anterior rotational instability necessarily leads to decompensation and early arthrosis. Since that is by no means the case and since total stability cannot be achieved in all cases either by primary or secondary stabilization operations, the indication for ligament reconstruction in fresh anterior cruciate ligament lesions in adults is an object of ongoing discussion. Secondary ligament reconstruction is indicated only if signs of decompensation have appeared. Patients without signs of decompensation following isolated anterior cruciate ligament rupture do not undergo ligament reconstruction but only follow a rehabilitation program [18]. Complicated injuries of the inner knee joint with extensive soft tissue or cartilaginous injuries continue to be treated primarily by means of ligament reconstruction in adults in order to restore the central pillar of stability.

If the physis is still open, this procedure is not practicable since most techniques in use would damage the growth plate adjacent to the knee joint to some extent. It must be kept in mind that the physis near the knee joint close relatively late which renders them vulnerable for a long time. Suture of an intraligamentous rupture in children and adolescents is as insufficient as in adults; this can also be seen from the results in our small group of patients. Partial ruptures may be satis-factorily cured conservatively with good stability, as also shown experimentally by Hefti in knee joints of growing rabbits [15, 33]. This is in accordance with the re-sults in one of our patients where a partial rupture was treated conservatively. A transosseous reinsertion of avulsed but intact ligaments seems to have a favour-able prognosis according to the literature and our own results [29, 33, 35]. It can be performed without endangering growth in the open physis. However, these lesions are rare. On the other hand the question arises whether full compensation of an instability following ligament reconstruction, ligamentous suture with and without augmentation or reinsertion is the direct result of specific aftercare and less the consequence of an operation [12]. Admittedly 15 of our patients exhibited a remaining instability on follow-up, but only one showed signs of decompen-sation. Moreover, two of our patients with complete loss of the cruciate ligaments do not exhibit signs of decompensation so far. In the literature no comments are given on this possibility either in adults or children, since it is basically assumed that only surgical treatment can establish favourable results.

Therefore differentiation not only between isolated and combined lesions, but also between lesions in open and closed physis is necessary for a decision about optimal diagnostic and therapeutic procedures. However, as in adults, we have to look for the presence and extent of associated injuries for the choice of primary treatment in lesions of the anterior cruciate ligaments as well as in eminence avul-sions in children [22, 37]. In any case, one should try for immediate reconstruction of the anterior cruciate ligament as the central pillar of stability in all combination injuries. This has to be achieved by reinsertion in open epiphyseal cartilages, pos-sibly combined with augmentation suture, and by ligament reconstruction with free transplantation of the patellar tendon in closed epiphyseal cartilages. In our opinion, however, primary reconstruction is not necessarily indicated in isolated lesions, unless there are pure avulsions in an otherwise intact ligament. To solve this question, the situation must be clarified arthroscopically in all children and adolescents presenting with primary haemarthrosis and positive Lachmann sign, but without radiological evidence of an osseous lesion, no matter whether the epi-physeal cartilages are open or closed, as long as we cannot safely determine the kind of lesion, its localization and relevant associated injuries by other methods, such as magnetic resonance imaging or computerized tomographic scanning [3, 8, 16, 19, 30, 37, 40]. In a fresh knee joint lesion the pivot shift sign seems to be primarily less indicative of a rupture of the cruciate ligaments than the Lachmann sign since pain might still be present [10, 26]. A positive Lachmann sign is a defi-nite indication for arthroscopy at our institution. If arthroscopy reveals an iso-lated, intraligamentous anterior rupture of the cruciate ligaments, we would, in the first instance, forego reconstruction of the ligaments in patients with open and closed physis. However, we would put these patients on restorative training as if we had performed ligament reconstruction. Subsequently, the patients may walk normally and take part in sports. Ligament reconstruction is indicated only if signs of decompensation occur n due course, in certain circumstances years later, since physis will have certainly closed by then. Following this procedure we do not think that there is a progressive evolution of osteoarthritis since osteoarthritis develops only after decompensated instability has persisted for years, but not in a compensated instability.

References

1. Bachelin P, Bugmann P (1988) Active subluxation in extension, radiological control in intercondylar eminence fractures in childhood. Z Kinderchir 43:180–182
2. Bartsch H (1987) Operative Behandlung der chronischen Kniebandinstabilität und Erfahrungen mit über 80 PTFE-TEX-Prothesen. Unfallheilkunde 189:971–975
3. Bergström R, Gillquist J (1984) Arthroscopy of the knee in children. J Pediatr Orthop 4: 542–545
4. Boszotta H, Sauer G, Ohrenberger G (1987) Zur Operationsindikation bei der chronischen vorderen Kniebandinstabilität. Unfallheilkunde 189:980–982
5. Bradley GW, Shives TC, Samuelson KM (1979) Ligament injuries in the knees of children. J Bone Joint Surg [A] June 61-A: 588–591
6. Clanton TO (1975) Knee ligament injuries in children. J Bone Joint Surg. Dec 61-A: 1195–1201
7. Dupont JY, Scellier C, Chaudières D (1986) Les lésions intra-articulaires et leur évolutivité au cours des ruptures récentes et anciennes du ligament croisé antérieur. Rapport préliminaire. Acta Orthop Belg 52 (4)
8. Eulenburg F, Gubba HH (1981) Zur Differentialdiagnose der Kniegelenksverletzung beim Kind und Jugendlichen. Orthop Prax 11:879–882
9. Fetto J, Marshall JL (1980) The natural history and diagnosis of anterior cruciate ligament insufficiency. Clin Orthop 147:29
10. Galway HR, MacIntosh DL (1980) The lateral pivot-shift: a symptom and sign of anterior cruciate ligament insufficiency. Clin Orthop 147:45
11. Gerber CH, Matter P (1983) Biomechanik des Kniegelenkes nach vorderer Kreuzbandruptur und dessen primärer Naht. In: Chapchal G (ed) Sportverletzungen und Sportschäden. Thieme, Stuttgart
12. Güssbacher A, Rompe G (1987) Das Muskelaufbautraining zur aktiven Gelenkstabilisation bei Kniebandinstabilitäten. Unfallheilkunde 189:991–993
13. Hackenbruch W, Kentsch A, Henche HR (1983) Diagnostik und Therapie der vorderen Rotationsinstabilität im Kniegelenk. In: Chapchal G (ed) Sportverletzungen und Sportschäden. Thieme, Stuttgart
14. Hassenpflug J, Blauth W, Rose D (1985) Zum Spannungsverhalten von Transplantaten zum Ersatz des vorderen Kreuzbandes. Unfallchirurg 88:151–158
15. Hefti F (1989) Natural healing of the anterior cruciate ligament. An experimental study. J Bone Joint Surg (to be published)
16. Henche HR, Hackenbruch W (1981) Die Arthroskopie beim traumatisierten kindlichen Kniegelenk. Orthop Prax 11:883–885
17. Hipp E, Gradinger R, Haw W, Ascherl R (1987) Vorderer Kreuzbandersatz mit Semitendinosussehne versus – freies Patellarsehnentransplantat. Unfallheilkunde 189:960–963
18. Holzach P, Hefti F, Gächter A (1986) Die vordere Kreuzbandplastik mit freiem Transplantat aus dem Ligamentum patellae. Unfallchirurg 89:176–182
19. Israel Z, Carroll NC (1982) The role of arthroscopy in children. J Pediatr Orthop 2:243–247
20. Jakob RP (1987) Indikation, Behandlung und Evaluation bei chronischer vorderer Kreuzband-Instabilität. Orthopade 16:130–139
21. Kiefer H, Claes L, Dürselen L (1987) Messungen zur vorderen Kniegelenksstabilität in Abhängigkeit von Muskelzug und alloplastischem Bandersatz. Unfallheilkunde 189:131–135
22. Lais E, Hertel P, Goudarzi AM (1987) Die arthroskopische Versorgung der dislozierten Ausrisse der Eminentia intercondylica bei Kindern und Jugendlichen. Unfallchirurgie 90:471–477

23. McDaniel WJ, Dameron DB (1983) The untreated anterior cruciate ligament rupture. Clin Orthop 172:158–163
24. Morrissy RT (1982) Arthroscopy of the knee in children. Clin Orthop 162:103
25. Mouret P, Zichner L (1987) Langzeitbeobachtungen von dynamischen Bandplastiken bei veralteter anteromedialer Rotationsinstabilität. Unfallheilk 189:987–991
26. Müller W (1982) Das Knie. Springer, Berlin Heidelberg New York
27. Nocak W, Schrf HP, Trepte CT (1987) Indikation, Technik und Ergebnisse der vorderen Kreuzbandnaht, der vorderen Kreuzbandsemitendinosusplastik und der C-Faser (Integraft) augmentierter Bandplastik. Unfallheilkunde 189:976–980
28. Noyes FR (1974) Biomechanics of anterior cruciate ligament failure: an analysis of strain rate sensitivity and mechanisms of failure in primates. J Bone Joint Surg [Am] 56-A:236–253
29. Odenstein M, Gillquist J (1984) Suture of fresh ruptures of the anterior cruciate ligament. A 5-year follow up. Acta Orthop Scand 55:270
30. Paar O, Reiser M, Bernett P, Riel KA (1983) Computertomogramm der Kreuzbänder als wichtigstes Hilfsmittel zur Diagnose von Sportverletzungen am Kniegelenk. In: Chapchal G (ed) Sportverletzungen und Sportschäden. Thieme, Stuttgart
31. Pässler HH, Stadler J, Berger R (1987) Erste Ergebnisse der operativen Behandlung von 200 veralteten Kreuzbandrupturen mit einem Kunststoffband (Stryker). Unfallheilkunde 189:963–971
32. Ramseier EW (1987) Häufigkeit und Spätresultate von Kreuzbandverletzungen am Kniegelenk. Unfallheilkunde 189:993–995
33. Sandberg R, Balkfors B (1987) Partial rupture of the anterior cruciate ligament, natural course. Clin Orthop 220:176
34. Schulheis KH, Kobler K, Helling HJ, Rehm KE (1987) Die operative Behandlung der chronischen Kniebandinstabilität. Unfallheilkunde 189:982–986
35. Strobel M, Stedtfeld HW, Stenzel H (1987) Pathomechanik der anteromedialen Rotationsinstabilität des Kniegelenkes in ihren verschiedenen Verletzungsgraden − leichenexperimentelle Studie. Unfallheilkunde 189:119–128
36. Tiling T, Schmid A, Edelmann M, Stadelmayer B (1987) Nachuntersuchungsergebnisse der freien und fettkörpergestielten Kreuzbandersatzplastiken. Unfallheilkunde 189:955–960
37. von Laer L, Brunner R (1984) Einteilung und Therapie der Ausrißfrakturen der Eminentia intercondylica im Wachstumsalter. Unfallheilkunde 87:144–150
38. Waldrop JI, Broussard S (1984) Disruption of the anterior cruciate ligament in a three-year-old child. J Bone Joint Surg [Am] 66-A (7):1113–1114
39. Wirth CJ (1983) Die differenzierte Therapie veralteter Kapselbandschäden am Kniegelenk und ihre Ergebnisse. In: Chapchal G (ed) Sportverletzungen und Sportschäden. Thieme, Stuttgart
40. Wirth CJ, Kolb M (1985) Hämarthros und "isolierte" vordere Kreuzbandläsion. Stellenwert der klinischen Diagnostik. Unfallchirurg 88:419–423

Treatment of Achalasia
by the Endoscopic-Pneumatic Dilatation Method

P. Dohrmann and W. Mengel

Summary

There is no definite cure for the loss of oesophageal peristalsis and incomplete relaxation of the lower oesophageal sphincter associated with achalasia. Pneumatic dilatation is a simple and safe method of achieving symptomatic improvement of the oesophageal passage. By this means five young patients became free of complaints within an average observation period of 6¾ years.

Zusammenfassung

Es gibt keine definitive Heilungsmöglichkeit des Verlusts der Ösophagusperistaltik und der inkompletten Erschlaffung des unteren Ösophagussphinkters bei der Achalasie. Die pneumatische Dilatation ist eine einfache und sichere Methode, eine symptomatische Besserung der Ösophaguspassage zu erzielen. Mit dieser Methode wurden 5 Kinder über einen durchschnittlichen Beobachtungszeitraum von 6¾ Jahren beschwerdefrei.

Résumé

Il est impossible d'obtenir une guérison définitive de la perte du péristaltisme oesophagien et du défaut de relaxation du sphincter de l'oesophage dans les cas d'achalasie. La dilatation pneumatique est une méthode simple et sûre pour obtenir une amélioration symptomatique du passage oesophagien. C'est ainsi que furent traités 5 enfants qui, suivis en moyenne pendant 6 ans et 9 mois, ne présentèrent plus de troubles.

Introduction

Achalasia is characterized by an incomplete relaxation of the oesophagogastric junction and a coincident disturbance of oesophageal motoricity. In the world literature the annual incidence is quoted at 1 case per 100000. Males and females are equally affected [12]. The disease can occur at any age, even in neonates [1–3, 7]; the proportion of children under 14 years of age, however, is at most 5% [10].

A neuromuscular disturbance of the autonomically innervated nonstriated muscles of the oesophagus is the pathophysiological cause. Although pathomorphological changes in the brain stem, in the vagal branches, in the plexus

Division of Paediatric Surgery, Department of Surgery, Christian Albrechts University Kiel, Arnold-Heller-Strasse 7, D-2300 Kiel, Federal Republic of Germany

Progress in Pediatric Surgery, Vol. 25
Angerpointner (Ed.)
© Springer-Verlag Berlin Heidelberg 1990

myentericus and in the nonstriated oesophageal muscles have been found, the pathogenesis has not yet been sufficiently explained [13].

Besides achalasia other terms are also used such as cardiospasm or idiopathic megaoesophagus. Nowadays the term achalasia is preferred because it describes the major functional disturbance in the act of swallowing, namely the complete relaxation of the lower oesophageal sphincter. It seems unlikely that achalasia is a congenital disease since, in most cases, it occurs late and is evenly distributed in the entire adult age group. Immediate proof that achalasia is an acquired disease is also lacking. Besides a possible autoimmunopathogenesis or a degenerative process most authors favour the hypothesis that neurotoxic damage to the nerve and ganglion cells plays a role in the genesis of achalasia. Treatment can consist of drug therapy, endoscopic or surgical procedures. The present study is a report on the endoscopic-pneumatic dilatation method.

Patients and Methods

From 1979 to 1981, five patients, 14–19 years of age, were treated for achalasia by endoscopic-pneumatic dilatation at the Kiel University Hospital. Based on clinical signs, achalasia was demonstrated by X-ray examination. The radiological findings were supplemented by endoscopy and manometry.

Dysphagia was the principal clinical sign, with almost all patients complaining of it. In the early stages dysphagia occurred irregularly and was intensified by emotional stress. Regurgitation of undigested food with large amounts of mucus was another almost obligate symptom. In some cases retrosternal pain occurred in the initial phase. Some patients suffered from cramp-like sensations which set in after a meal or during the night. Contrast radiography of the oesophagus showed uncoordinated motility with a loss of propulsive oesophageal contractions and a constant constriction of the gastrooesophageal junction, i.e. of the lower oesophageal sphincter.

Staging was done according to Postlethwait [8], the radiological findings serving as a basis. The three types are classified as flask, fusiform and sigmoid (Fig. 1).

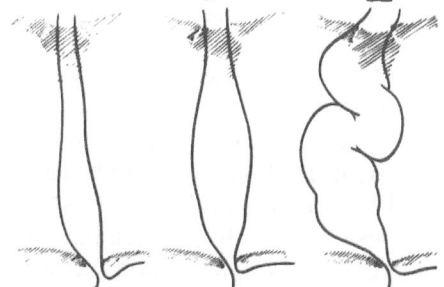

Fig. 1. Radiological staging of achalasia according to Postlethwait [8].
I flask; II fusiform; III sigmoid

Table 1. Data and characteristics of the achalasia patients

Patient	Age at diagnosis (years)	Sex	Duration of illness (years)	Radiological staging according to Postlethwait [8]	Symptoms	Loss of weight[a]
1	17	F	0.5	I	Dysphagia, pain	−
2	15	M	5.0	I	Dysphagia	−
3	19	M	1.0	II	Dysphagia, aspiration	+
4	16	F	2.0	II	Dysphagia	−
5	14	M	5.0	I	Dysphagia	−

[a] + weight gain; − weight loss

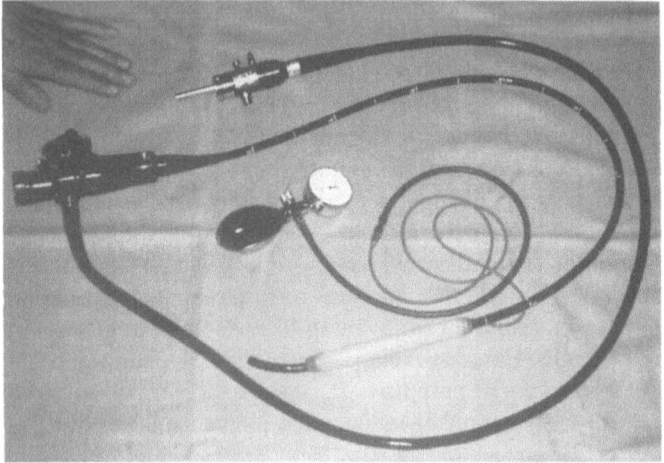

Fig. 2. Dilatation balloon with manometer attached to an Olympus P3 endoscope

The staging of the five patients was as follows: three cases of stage I and two cases of stage II (Table 1).

A paediatric endoscope (Olympus P3) was used for the endoscopic-pneumatic dilatation. A special balloon was attached about 20 cm proximal to the tip of the device (Fig. 2). This dilatation balloon consists of a soft silicone tube measuring 15 cm in length and a closely fitting inflatable rubber balloon that is reinforced at the ends with metal rings and contained within a fabric balloon lined with rubber.

After insertion of the endoscope, the dilatation balloon is placed in the cardia and its position is checked by inverting the optics. One-third of the balloon must be visible (Fig. 3). Dilatation is done under permanent visual inspection; thus, the position of the balloon can be corrected. The balloon is then inflated in this fixed position as quickly as possible to the specified diameter of 5 cm (300 mm Hg) and

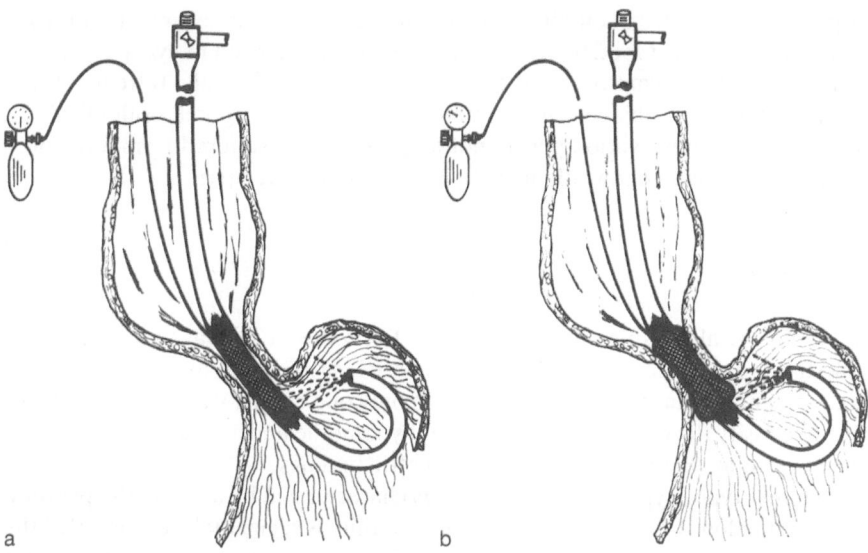

Fig. 3a, b. Endoscopic-pneumatic dilatation. **a** Introduction of the dilatation balloon and checking position by inversion of the optics, **b** during dilatation with visual inspection

it is kept under pressure for 1 min. An inspection of the cardia and the oesophagus when removing the gastroscope and a survey radiograph of the thorax complete the procedure. This method of treatment requires neither hospitalization nor anaesthesia.

Results

Five patients, 14–19 years of age, were treated by the endoscopic-pneumatic dilatation method. A single dilatation was sufficient in four cases. One girl had to be treated four times before there was an improvement. Follow-up was done in all cases and the therapeutic success was checked by anamnesis, X-rays and endo-

Table 2. Results of achalasia by endoscopic-pneumatic dilatation

Patient	Symptom-free period (years)	Number of dilatations	Complications	Clinical success
1	8½	4	None	Good
2	6½	1	None	Very good
3	6½	1	None	Good
4	6¼	1	None	Very good
5	6	1	None	Very good

scopy. The period between dilatation and the last follow-up examination ranged from 5 to 8½ years. Good to very good results were achieved in every case.

Freedom from symptoms was considered a very good result. Infrequent dysphagia without any subjective impairment was classified as a good result (Table 2). Over the entire observation period not a single patient suffered from a renewed onset of complaints that would have to be considered a relapse.

Discussion

The radiological classification according to Postlethwait [8] was used in the present study to determine the stages of achalasia. At the time the diagnoses were made a manometric study had been done in only one case, it was therefore impossible to classify the cases into hypermotile, hypomotile and amotile [9] as is generally done today on the basis of the manometric findings.

The first type, hypermotile achalasia, is characterized by a rise in the pressure at rest of the lower oesophageal sphincter. Motility is segmental, relaxation of the distal oesophageal sphincter is incomplete, residual pressure is low. It is difficult or virtually impossible to diagnose this form by radiology or endoscopy. Normal or insignificantly raised pressure at rest of the lower oesophageal sphincter, incomplete or premature deglutition reflex relaxation, increased residual pressure and segmental hypotonic oesophageal peristalsis are associated with the most frequent form, namely hypermotile achalasia. Radiological and endoscopic studies reveal a dilated oesophagus with delayed passage of the contrast medium in the region of the cardia. The final stage of this disease is called amotile achalasia. This type is virtually unknown in children or adolescents. X-rays reveal a grotesquely dilated oesophagus coiled like a corkscrew; peristalsis is generally normal and deglutition reflex relaxation is absent (stage III according to Postlethwait).

The aim of every method of treatment is a symptomatic improvement of the insufficient relaxation of the distal oesophageal sphincter. A true cure, i.e. restoring the physiological oesophageal motoricity is impossible. Besides drug treatment with glucagon and nitro preparations, which aims at improving subjective complaints and has been quite effective to date, there are nowadays two other competing procedures for treating achalasia: myotomy is a surgical approach whereas dilatation with so-called balloon dilators is a conservative one.

Since 1978 endoscopic-pneumatic dilatation has been the treatment of choice for established achalasia at the Kiel University Hospital. Definite diagnosis is based on the systematic investigation of the length, on the history, on subjective complaints, such as dysphagia, regurgitation, pain and heartburn, and on radiological and endoscopic examination.

It is hardly possible to compare clinical results because of the small number of cases (incidence 2% –8% [8]) and also because various authors have used different therapeutic approaches. Basically, a gastro-oesophageal reflux tends to develop more often after a myotomy [12] than following a dilatation. Some try to optimize this by a Nissen fundoplication [6], others by a less extensive myotomy [4]. Some authors recommend a step-by-step procedure [13] in order to achieve optimum results while performing the dilatation, whereas others favour a rather rapid inflation of the balloon [11]. The numerous procedures underline the uncertainty regarding the correct procedure.

If one assumes that the aetiology of achalasia is unclear, that the disease has a progressive character [5] and that only symptomatic improvement can be achieved by every reported procedure, then the treatment of choice should initially be the least extensive and the least stressful procedure.

By means of the present method five young patients, aged 14–19 years, became free of complaints over an average observation period of 6¾ years. Compared with an operative approach this method is less stressful and less risky and does not preclude surgical intervention at a later stage. The procedure therefore seems indicated in primary therapy for established achalasia.

References

1. Asch MJ, Liebmann W, Lachmann RS, Moore TC (1972) Esophageal achalasia. J Pediatr Surg 9:911–912
2. Eaton H (1972) Achalasia of the cardia in a three-month-old infant treated successfully by a modified Heller's operation. Aust N Z J Surg 41:240–244
3. Elder JB (1970) Achalasia of the cardia in childhood. Digestion 3:90–96
4. Elli HF, Gibbs PS, Crozier RE (1980) Esophagomyotomy for achalasia of the esophagus. Ann Surg 192:157–161
5. Imdahl H (1981) Diskussionsbemerkung: Symposium Aktuelle Chirurgie, Berlin
6. Koch A, Bettex M, Tschäppeler H, König W (1938) Die Funktion des Oesophagus nach Kardiomyotomie bei der kindlichen Achalasie. Z Kinderchir 38:206–210
7. Magilner AD, Isard HJ (1971) Achalasia of the esophagus in infancy. Radiology 98:81–82
8. Postlethwait RW (1979) Surgery of the esophagus. Appleton-Century-Crofts, New York, pp 77–117
9. Siewert JR, Lepsien G (1982) Klassifikation und Differentialdiagnose der Achalasie. In: Häring R (ed) Oesophaguschirurgie. Edition Medizin, Weinheim, pp 41–46
10. Tachovsky TJ, Lynn HB, Ellis FH (1968) The surgical approach to esophageal achalasia in children. J Pediatr Surg 3:226–231
11. Troidl H, Vestweber KH, Sommer H (1980) Neues Verfahren zur pneumatischen Dehnung bei der Achalasie mit dem flexiblen Endoskop. In: Abstracts of the IVth European congress of gastrointestinal endoscopy. Thieme, Stuttgart, p 24
12. Vantrappen G, Hellemanns J (1974) Motility disturbances of the esophagus. Achalasia. In: Vantrappen G, Hellemans J (eds) Diseases of the esophagus. Springer, Berlin Heidelberg New York, pp 287–354 (Handbuch der inneren Medizin, 5th edn, vol 3/1)
13. Wienbeck M (1976) Achalasie. In: Siewert R, Blum AL, Waldeck F (eds) Funktionsstörungen der Speiseröhre. Springer, Berlin Heidelberg New York, pp 154–182

Subject Index

Progress in Pediatric Surgery

Volume 24

J. Yokoyama, Keio University, Tokyo;
T. A. Angerpointner, University of Munich (Eds.)

Constipation and Fecal Incontinence and Motility Disturbances of the Gut

1989. Approx. 240 pp. 113 figs. Hardcover
ISBN 3-540-50813-9

This volume has been authored by internationally reputed experts from Japan and Europe and reflects the state of the art in the field of pediatric surgery.

The first section on constipation and incontinence shows the fast pace of research in Japan on the subject. In particular, pathophysiological studies have led to improved diagnostic techniques and the clinical application of anorectal manometry.

The second section discusses a topic that has long been of great interest: motility disturbances of the gut. New insights from improved diagnostic methods, pathophysiology and histology have induced new therapeutic trials and a better understanding of diseases such as Hirschsprung's disease and neuronal intestinal dysplasia.

Despite the many recent improvements, much clinical and experimental work remains to be done to resolve these problems.

Springer-Verlag Berlin
Heidelberg New York London
Paris Tokyo Hong Kong

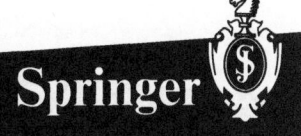

Springer

Progress in Pediatric Surgery

Volume 23

L. Spitz, London; **P. Wurnig,** Vienna;
T. A. Angerpointner, Munich (Eds.)

Surgery in Solitary Kidney and Corrections of Urinary Transport Disturbances

1989. VIII, 205 pp. 136 figs. 34 tabs. Hardcover
ISBN 3-540-50485-0

Volume 22

L. Spitz, London; **P. Wurnig,** Vienna;
T. A. Angerpointner, Munich (Eds.)

Pediatric Surgical Oncology

1989. VIII, 180 pp. 78 figs. 44 tabs. Hardcover
ISBN 3-540-17769-8

Volume 21

P. Wurnig, Vienna (Ed.)

Trachea and Lung Surgery in Childhood

1987. X, 147 pp. 75 figs. Hardcover ISBN 3-540-17232-7

Volume 20

P. P. Rickham, Zurich (Ed.)

Historical Aspects of Pediatric Surgery

1986. X, 285 pp. 119 figs. Hardcover ISBN 3-540-15960-6

Volume 19

P. Wurnig, Vienna (Ed.)

Long-gap Esophageal Atresia Prenatal Diagnosis of Congenital Malformations

1986. XII, 205 pp. 86 figs. Hardcover ISBN 3-540-15881-2

Springer-Verlag Berlin
Heidelberg New York London
Paris Tokyo Hong Kong

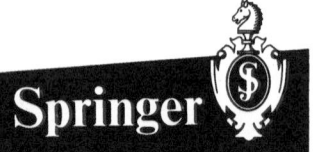

Springer